MANUAL OF
DEVELOPMENTAL
DIAGNOSIS

Hilda Knobloch, M.D., Dr. P.H.

Medical Specialist, Eleanor Roosevelt Developmental Services
N.Y. State Office of Mental Retardation and Developmental Disabilities
Professor of Pediatrics
Head, Division of Developmental Disabilities
Department of Pediatrics
Albany Medical College of Union University
Albany, New York

In Collaboration with Frances Stevens, M.S.

Research Associate, Department of Pediatrics
Albany Medical College of Union University
Albany, New York

With Assistance from Anthony F. Malone, M.D.

Medical Specialist, Eleanor Roosevelt Developmental Services
Assistant Professor, Department of Pediatrics
Albany Medical College of Union University
Albany, New York

Harper & Row, Publishers
Hagerstown

Cambridge
New York
Philadelphia
San Francisco

London
Mexico City
São Paulo
Sydney

1817

MANUAL OF DEVELOPMENTAL DIAGNOSIS

*The Administration and Interpretation
of the
Revised Gesell and Amatruda
Developmental and Neurologic Examination*

MANUAL OF DEVELOPMENTAL DIAGNOSIS: The Administration and Interpretation of the Revised Gesell and Amatruda Developmental and Neurologic Examination. Copyright © 1980 by Harper & Row, Publishers, Inc. All rights reserved. Printed in the United States of America. For information address Medical Department, Harper & Row Publishers, Inc., 2350 Virginia Avenue, Hagerstown, Maryland 21740.

Library of Congress Cataloging in Publication Data

Knobloch, Hilda, DATE
   Manual of developmental diagnosis.
   Based on Gesell and Amatruda's Developmental diagnosis.
   Bibliography
   Includes index.
   1. Child development—Testing. 2. Child development deviations—Diagnosis. I. Stevens, Frances M., joint author. II. Malone, Anthony F., joint author. III. Gesell, Arnold Lucius, 1880–1961. Gesell and Amatruda's Developmental diagnosis. IV. Title. [DNLM: 1. Child development. 2. Child development deviations. WS350 K714m]
RJ51.D48K58   618.92′8588075   80-14833
ISBN 0-06-141437-9

1   3   5   7   6   4   2

Contents

Preface

Arnold Gesell and his gifted clinician collaborator, Catherine Amatruda, made fundamental contributions to the understanding and assessment of infant and child neuropsychologic development. Their methods as clinical tools in infant neuropsychiatry have withstood the test of time and have demonstrated the validity of clinically oriented infant assessment for predicting future development as well as for immediate treatment and intervention.

After the untimely death of Dr. Amatruda and the later death of Dr. Gesell, Benjamin Pasamanick and I revised their basic clinical text, *Developmental Diagnosis.** We tempered their emphasis on innate maturational processes by stressing more firmly the social context in which the biologic factors operate. We provided the long-term procedures of testing reliability and validity that their short experience with clinical applications, derived from years of normative research, could not produce. We added much of the new scientific information of the intervening 30-odd years since the first edition, as well as data from our own clinical and research activities, and meshed our ideas with the elegant language and conceptualizations of our two teachers.

As we had pointed out in the third edition, our examinations of thousands of infants and children in different settings, since the original schedules were delineated, indicated that the rate of maturation had accelerated, but trends of development, interrelationships and integrations had not altered to any significant degree. Lacking a systematic investigation, it was not possible to make arbitrary changes on the basis of clinical hunches; therefore we did not alter the developmental schedules.

*Knobloch H, Pasamanick B (eds): Gesell and Amatruda's Developmental Diagnosis, 3rd ed. Hagerstown, Harper & Row, 1974

The present Manual is the outcome of the examination of over 1000 infants and children at 20 different ages ranging from 4 weeks to 36 months, which now permits age-placement of behavior patterns to reflect current development. The actual changes are not too different from what the clinical hunches, based on the examination of 1000 40-week olds in the 1952 Study of Prematures,* suggested they might be. The shifts that have occurred range from a 5% acceleration in fine motor behavior in some of the older ages to 16% and 17% in the personal-social and gross motor behaviors. Some illustrations are shown in Appendix A, and the details can be garnered from the schedules themselves in Chapter 3.

We have no neuroanatomic or biochemical evidence as firm documentation of significant structural changes; we would not expect any. However, we do have epidemiologic data from the increased survival of and the decreased incidence of neuropsychiatric disability in very low birth weight infants to indicate that the amount of central nervous system *damage* has decreased. We have suggestive evidence from these same infants† that the improvement is the result of the improved maternal and prenatal status to a large extent.

The continuing failure to demonstrate, in the absence of neurologic dysfunction, behavioral differences in infancy and early toddlerhood on the basis of sociocultural status lends credence to the concept that the acceleration that has occurred has a biologic and not a psychologic basis. It is the result of the improvement in health, consumer sophistication, and economic status that is consequent to an affluent society, advances that have trickled down to all but its most impoverished members. This progress is a post-World War II, and not a recent, phenomenon. Whether it will continue in our current post-Vietnam War era of retrenchment and recession remains to be seen.

We are presenting the material as a manual in order to bring together in relatively compact form the information needed for the administration and interpretation of the Revised Gesell and Amatruda Developmental and Neurologic Examination. We have not quite met our goal of a pocket manual, but we have come close. The bulk of the

*Knobloch H, Pasamanick B: An evaluation of the consistency and predictive value of the 40-week Gesell developmental schedule. In Shagass C, Pasamanick B (eds): Child Development and Child Psychiatry. Psychiatric Research Reports 13. Washington, Am Psych Assn, 1960, pp 10–31

†Malone A, Knobloch H, Stevens F, Ellison P, Risemberg H: Problems assessing outcome of neonatal intensive care. Unpublished data, 1977

material consists of the revised Gesell Developmental Schedules with their accompanying narrative descriptions for the key ages, and their glossaries. There are two chapters on the conduct of the examination and the specifics of the examination procedures. Included also are the two screening procedures, the revised Developmental Screening Inventory and the revised Parent Developmental Questionnaire based on the schedules. These are the bare bones on which a discussion of the administration and interpretation of the developmental neurologic examination is built.

The Manual stands alone in its presentation of the revised developmental stages and the collation of the various facets of the examination technique into a compact form. But it adheres strictly to *Developmental Diagnosis*, substituting the new material appropriately and making modifications where indicated. The minimal amount of clinical material necessary for some appreciation of developmental deviations has been extracted from *Developmental Diagnosis*, in some cases wholesale. Dr. Pasamanick provided the historical and scientific insights which enabled the revised third edition to reflect broader social horizons. In that edition, we have emphasized the neurologic and sociocultural material and the scientific advances of the recent decades. But we continue to owe a great debt to our two teachers who were the pioneer investigators in early child development and the neurology of infancy. *Developmental Diagnosis* is an essential companion piece and should be referred to at every turn.

While diagnosis remains within the province of the physician, and in the case of developmental deviations within the province of the developmental diagnostician, we believe this manual will be useful to the many professionals who work with children: general practitioners, pediatricians, neurologists, psychiatrists, nurses, physical, occupational and speech therapists, psychologists, social workers and teachers.

We wish to encourage the use of the materials within this volume. Professionals engaged in the evaluation and care of infants and young children may reproduce the developmental schedules and the other forms used for developmental evaluation without requesting the permission of either Harper & Row or the authors of this book, provided that the use is for nonprofit purposes and the authors and source of the material are acknowledged properly. As an alternative, the forms may be purchased at cost from the authors.

The examination materials necessary for carrying out the evaluation can be obtained on a commercial basis from Mr. Nigel Cox, 69 Fawn Drive, Cheshire, CT 06410.

H.K.

Acknowledgments

So many have contributed in some way to the production of this Manual that we cannot mention them all. It was a grant from the Johnson and Johnson Institute for Pediatric Service, secured through the offices of Horace Hodes, M.D., that enabled us to start this 5-year project. A generous contribution from the Esther A. and Joseph Klingenstein Fund, Inc., obtained with the assistance of Harold Williams, enabled us to complete it.

Richard Martin, computer programmer, put our initial clinical data into manageable form for analysis. Michael Fabrizio, M.D., during his fellowship year with the Division of Developmental Disabilities, and a host of pediatric residents, medical students and other volunteers, helped in coding, transcribing and collating the data.

Among the diverse succession of secretarial assistants we must mention four: Danette Odom Dergosits and Janice Coffey who worked during the three years of data collection; Gail Connors who typed the bulk of the manuscript so neatly; and Lidia Minicuci, who did all the odds and ends, put the finishing touches on the manuscript and caught our editing oversights.

Pat Murphy Carrasco drew the illustrations for Chapter 3, and Noel Carrasco, M.D., devised the safety pin task to help fill in the gap in fine motor behavior that exists at the older ages.

Most of all we owe a debt to the parents of the children who participated so enthusiastically and made it all possible.

MANUAL OF
DEVELOPMENTAL
DIAGNOSIS

1
Developmental Assessment

Developmental assessment is essentially a device for determining the integrity and functional maturity of the child's nervous system. The clinician is interested in the individual as a whole—in the total integrated functioning and behavior at all stages of development, in the context of society and its institutions.

The physician is concerned with the maturity and health of an infant or child; he has the responsibility for making a diagnosis, even if it is one of no disease. In his role as developmental diagnostician, he is not asked to derive an IQ, or measure "intelligence" as such. It is his task to assess central nervous system function: to identify the presence of any neuromotor or sensory deficit, to discover the existence of treatable developmental disorders, to detect infants at risk of subsequent deterioration, and to determine pathologic conditions of the brain which preclude normal intellectual function, no matter how optimal the environmental circumstances.

BEHAVIOR AND BEHAVIORAL DEVELOPMENT

Behavior is rooted in the brain and in the sensory and motor systems. It is subject to diagnosis because it is an orderly process. Behavior patterns are not whimsical or accidental by-products. The timing, smoothness, and integration at one age foretell behavior at a later age. The human fetus becomes the human infant; the human infant, the human child and adult. This orderly sequence represents the human genetic endowment. The behavioral end-products of the devel-

1

opmental process are a consequence of continuing reciprocal interaction between genetic endowment and the environment.

Behavior develops. Normal behavior assumes characteristic patterns as it develops. The principles and practice of developmental diagnosis rest on these simple far-reaching propositions. Developmental diagnosis consists of a discriminating observation of behavior patterns and their appraisal by comparison with normal behavior patterns. A normal behavior pattern is a criterion of maturity which has been defined by systematic studies of the average healthy course of behavioral development. Study of thousands of healthy infants and young children has ascertained the average trends of their behavioral development. The sequences of development (*i.e.,* the order in which behavior patterns appear), and the chronologic age at which each pattern appears, are significantly uniform. Of course, note is taken of the ranges of individual variation, but these variations cling closely to a central mean. With few exceptions, the term *normal* is used in its connotation of *healthy* in this volume.

THE FUNCTION OF DEVELOPMENTAL ASSESSMENT

Behavioral tests have the same logic as any of the functional tests of clinical neurology. They are designed to establish normality, to reveal even minor deviations in relatively healthy children, and to define the maturity and integrity of the central nervous system. However, behavioral observation always must be supplemented by adequate social and medical history and appropriate laboratory investigations.

Since most of the defects and diseases of infancy and early childhood are not localized lesions occurring in an already mature central nervous system, the areas of dysfunction are not revealed by standard adult neurologic examinations. Therefore, behavioral evaluation may be more competent in disclosing significant lesions, defects, distortions, and retardations in the organization of the developing nervous system.

The situations of the developmental evaluation bring out characteristic reactions, at specific ages, which would not be forthcoming at all using more artificial procedures. Behavioral assessments in each of the five major areas open the infant to opportunistic observation. They call into play his organs of vision, hearing, touch, and proprioception. They make a wide range of demands upon motor coordination, and inevitably call into requisition the higher cortical controls. For these reasons, they comprise both a maturity assessment and a neuromotor and sensory examination, and permit differentiation and detailed exploration of both normal and abnormal responses.

The developmental, neuromotor, and sensory objectives of this evaluation cannot be divorced. The infant's behavior must be surveyed and appraised in terms of his true chronologic age. This behavior may prove normal, it may show general retardation in maturation, or it may show deviations which are so distinctive that they point to faults in neural structure or to impairments in central nervous system integration. There are no right or wrong behavioral responses, or successes or failures, because the examination is concerned with the infant's behavioral status. Any response in behavior is appropriate to some age or level of central nervous system function.

THE DEVELOPMENTAL DIAGNOSIS OF BEHAVIOR

THE FIVE FIELDS OF BEHAVIOR

A single behavior pattern, such as prying with the index finger, may have a high degree of diagnostic import. However, the human organism is a complicated action system; adequate developmental diagnosis requires examination of the quality and integration of five fields of behavior, each representing a different aspect of development. These five major fields are (1) adaptive behavior, (2) gross motor behavior, (3) fine motor behavior, (4) language behavior, and (5) personal-social behavior.

Adaptive Behavior, the most important field, is concerned with the organization of stimuli, the perception of relationships, the dissection of wholes into their component parts, and the reintegration of these parts in a meaningful fashion. Included in this field are finer sensorimotor adjustments to objects and situations: the coordination of eyes and hands in reaching and manipulation; the ability to utilize motor equipment appropriately in the solution of practical problems; the capacity to initiate new adjustments in the presence of simple problem situations. Significant behavior patterns will be displayed even in an infant's exploitation of a simple object such as a hand bell. He will reveal growing resourcefulness. Adaptive behavior is the forerunner of later "intelligence," which utilizes previous experience in the solution of new problems.

Gross Motor Behavior includes postural reactions, head balance, sitting, standing, creeping, and walking.

Fine Motor Behavior consists of the use of the hands and fingers in the prehensory approach to, grasping, and manipulation of an object.

Each field of motor behavior is of special interest to the physician because it has so many neurologic implications. The motor capacities of a child constitute a natural starting point for an estimate of his maturity; however, too often they constitute the only parameters which are evaluated. Motor and adaptive behavior—in fact, all forms of behavior—are intimately interrelated, but they can and must be separated in diagnostic usage.

Language Behavior likewise assumes distinctive patterns which furnish clues to the organization of the child's central nervous system. The term is used broadly to include all visible and audible forms of communication, whether by facial expression, gesture, postural movements, vocalizations, words, phrases, or sentences. Language behavior, moreover, includes mimicry and comprehension of the communications of others. Articulate speech is a function which depends upon a social milieu, but which also requires the readiness of sensorimotor and cortical structures. Preverbal phases prepare for the verbal phases. Inarticulate vocalizations and vocal signs precede words, which are learned from and reinforced by others in the environment. The underlying stages, in the absence of distorting neurologic or environmental factors, are as orderly as those observed in the fields of adaptive and motor behavior.

Personal-Social Behavior comprises the child's personal reactions to the social culture in which he lives. These reactions are so multitudinous, variegated, and contingent upon environment that they might seem to be beyond the reach of developmental diagnosis. But as in the other four fields, these behavior patterns are determined by intrinsic growth factors. Bladder and bowel control, for example, are cultural requirements, shaped by social demands, but their attainment depends upon the child's neuromotor maturity. This relationship holds for many of the child's abilities and attitudes: feeding abilities, self-dependence in play, cooperation, and responsiveness to training and social conventions. Even though personal-social behavior is particularly subject to societal goals and individual variations, the variations have normal limits and diagnostic implications.

ORGANIZATIONAL ASPECTS

These five areas of behavior form the basic fabric of his behavior repertoire, but *equally important is how* he demonstrates his developmental maturity. Are his sensory modalities of sight, hearing, and touch intact? If he has motor or sensory handicaps, has he developed alternate pathways for the expression of his comprehension of the world? How organized and integrated are his responses, his attention, and his discrimination? Is he thoughtful, or impulsive and haphazard? Are his emotional responses stable or fragile? Are they appropriate to the situation and his age? What is his level of tolerance to frustration?

Even though intimate interrelationships exist among the different facets of behavioral development, each aspect demands separate analysis and study for adequate differential diagnosis and prognosis. They cannot be summed and averaged. However, all are evaluated concurrently in the course of the developmental assessment. The child cannot be fragmented into psychometric and neurologic halves, or into any other independent subdivisions. Neuromotor and sensory integrity and maturational status are inextricably intertwined. In Chapter 5, six broad aspects of neuropsychiatric disability will be discussed in more detail: (1) intellectual potential, (2) neuromotor status, (3) seizure disorders, (4) sensory impairment, (5) qualitative and integrative aspects, and (6) specific syndromes.

AGE AND ASSESSMENT

Because of the generally amorphous character of neonatal behavior, diagnosis and prediction of cortical integrity from this period of life are not possible. Responses at 1 and 4 weeks of age are essentially similar; even at 4 weeks, the infant's behavior has validity only for gross abnormality and group predictiveness related to high risk factors, such as low birth weight or intracranial hemorrhage. Not until the virtually complete release from the domination of the tonic-neck-reflex by 16 weeks does adaptive behavior indicate the cortical intactness predictive of later behavior. This initial crudity is replaced by greater precision with time, and 28 weeks is an opportune time for early detection of developmental delays. The optimal period for evaluation for research purposes is 40 weeks, when all parts of the body have come under some degree of voluntary control, and compensation for minor disabilities has not yet occurred. In the first year of life, behavior is for the most part uninfluenced by social environmental factors and is dependent primarily on the intactness of the infant's central nervous system—unless the environmental factors are grossly deviant, such as starvation or marked malnutrition, abuse, dysstimulation, or institutionalization.

PREDICTION FROM INFANT ASSESSMENT

The predictive value of infant examinations for later development hinges on what the purpose of the evaluation is considered to be. If a healthy cerebral cortex is demonstrated in infancy by a normal tempo, quality, and integration of behavioral development, cortical integrity will continue to be normal provided there are no intercurrent noxious events. Performance can be depressed by biologic factors leading to organic disease of the brain or by social and psychologic factors resulting from adverse environmental circumstances. On the other hand, acceleration in developmental rate can only result from learning in an enriched and stimulating sociocultural milieu.

Clear delineation of what is expected from clinical diagnoses in infancy is essential. First is the identification of the subnormal infant with organic disease of the brain which precludes normal development, even under optimal circumstances. Next is the differentiation of primarily neuromotor and sensory handicaps from intellectual handicaps. In addition, there is the ascertainment of diseases and environmental factors which may depress developmental rates, particularly those factors amenable to treatment. On the basis of his performance as an infant, the individual without organic disease of the central nervous system, who later will be culturally retarded, cannot be detected. Neither is it clinically important, nor generally possible, to identify the infant who later will be superior because of exposure to increased opportunities for learning, except by using nonbehavioral indices such as parental status. In the *undamaged infant*, the parents' sociocultural level is a better index of later performance on a standard intelligence test than is the infant DQ.

Clinicians would be satisfied with the following statement: This infant has no central nervous system impairment, and his intellectual potential is within the normal range; depending on his life experiences between now and school age, at that time he will have a Stanford-Binet IQ that is average or above, unless qualitative changes in the central nervous system are caused by noxious agents, or unless gross changes in milieu alter major variables of function.

Predictions are much more precise than this clinically acceptable statement. Longitudinal data from several studies[1] of infants define the contributions made by infant intellectual potential and neuromotor status to later function, and identify several factors that modify the course of development and the direction in which they do so. The literature on the subject emphasizes numerical correlations; such correlations are not the most important aspects of development to examine. In school-age children without organic impairment, tests of intelligence have limited usefulness as indices of the validity of infant developmental examination methods. Errors of clinical application will be avoided if we remember that the DQ and IQ refer only to the end products of development. In themselves, they do not take into account the etiologies of defects and deviations, the medical history of the child, the presence of specific disabilities, and differences in environmental and experiential factors.

2
The Conduct of the Evaluation

The conduct of a developmental diagnostic assessment and the beginning of management entails five steps: (1) a history and preliminary interview, (2) the formal behavioral examination, in an established order, (3) recording of the results and a diagnostic review of the evaluation as a whole, (4) a discussion of the findings and recommendations with the parents, and (5) a written report for the child's record and for the referring source. This chapter provides a general discussion of these five tasks and includes procedural details. Sample forms are given in Chapter 6.

Some sections of this chapter have pertinence primarily for the consultant specialist in developmental diagnosis; for such situations the assumption is made that the examination represents the first contact with the family. Detailed information may or may not be available from the referring physician or agency, but the general nature of the problem is known.

HISTORY AND PRELIMINARY INTERVIEW

As in all of medicine, an adequate history is a *sine qua non* for diagnosis. It is essential to obtain this information, preferably before examining the child. An adequate history includes information about the family, the specific pregnancy, labor, delivery and neonatal period, illnesses, convulsive seizures, past development, current behavior, and pertinent environmental and social variables. The physician providing continuous care for a child should have this information already at hand.

For the consultant, foreknowledge about the child should be gained by sending the appropriate Revised Parent Developmental Questionnaire to the parents prior to an appointment (see Chapter 7). For infants under 18 months of age, these questions will focus on behavior appropriate to the child's age; for children over 18 months they should cover some details of past development also. The information obtained in this manner can be transferred to the appropriate developmental schedules prior to the child's arrival.

Whenever possible, the appointment should be scheduled for the time of day which coincides with the child's period of greatest alertness and cooperation. The replies from the parents and their chief complaint will be clues to the complexity of the ensuing evaluation. Obtaining the needed additional history and the behavioral examination generally can be combined in a single session. If a child is restless, or the history extremely involved, the child can be removed by one parent while the other is being interviewed or, less desirably, the examination can be conducted first.

The interview should be friendly and informal rather than inquisitorial. On the other hand, little is gained and much lost by open-ended generalities. The questions should be specific enough so that there is no confusion in the parents' minds about the information being requested. Often it will be helpful if the examiner illustrates what he means. Each examiner formulates questions in his own way, of course—the answer to one question often changing the form of the next. Rigid adherence to a standard form is neither expected nor desirable, but systematic review is vital.

The information should be recorded as it is elicited. Any necessary clarification of the replies about behavior already received from the parents follows, and information about items not included on the questionnaire sent them is added to what has been transcribed already to developmental schedules. Obviously, the entire age range of behavior patterns is not covered. The examiner uses the information he has obtained already and the child's behavior he may have observed during the interview to modify his questions.

The general approach in asking the parents about behavior patterns is to cover one area of behavior at a time, exploring the upper limits in one field before proceeding to the next. Inquiry is made systematically about gross motor, language, and personal-social behavior; questions about adaptive and fine motor areas may be curtailed, since these abilities generally are exhibited by the child in the course of the examination. On each of the developmental schedules presented in

Chapter 3, certain items in the history columns have been blocked out, indicating that these patterns are so precisely defined that the behavior must be observed by the examiner.

In all instances, the decision about the need for additional information on past development can be made by asking two questions to supplement the parents' chief complaint and concerns: *"Has your child ever failed to make progress?" "Has he ever lost any behavior once acquired?"*

A word of caution is necessary about the reliability of the history obtained. It is extremely important to believe what the parents are telling you; parents are good observers of their child's behavior, and they do not come to you with intent to deceive. The burden of proof that they are wrong is on you, and you will get into far more difficulties in diagnosis if you discount their reports. If what the parents say is at variance with your initial impression of the child or knowledge of developmental patterns, make certain that they understand the questions you are asking and that you are asking them correctly, or look for some modifying factors. For example, the mother of a 28-week-old may tell you that he is able to sit leaning forward on his hands for support, but when you ask about his head control, she says, "It's terrible, doctor." Your immediate reaction is to say she is an inadequate historian, because it isn't possible at this age for the infant to support himself in sitting and yet have poor head control. However, when you see an akinetic seizure, with loss not only of head control but of all body control, her answers are understandable. You have not been specific enough in your interrogation.

With practice, the examiner will become familiar enough with the area of developmental diagnosis so that his attention will not be glued to the forms. He will be able to listen to what the parents are saying; he will not repeat questions for which information already has been given spontaneously; and he will be able to look at the child and the parents for important clues their impromptu behavior may provide. However, *the examiner must be alert to the child's state, and should interrupt the questioning and proceed to the behavioral evaluation if excessive restlessness supervenes.* How the child tolerates the interview and what he does during it have diagnostic significance in themselves.

Rapport with the child should be established during the interview, before beginning the examination. This rapport is facilitated if the examiner wears a coat of a color other than the white usually associated with a doctor. If an infant is sensitive to strangers, or if a child is wary, it is good policy to delay any direct overtures to the young visitor and give chief attention to the mother. This seeming neglect will in itself tend to disarm the child. He will conclude that the examiner has no violent designs upon him, and as confidence takes root, *you may tentatively offer him a toy during the course of the questioning. If he does not accept the proffer, he needs more time to make his initial adjustment. When he accepts the toy freely from your hands, he has accepted you. Then it usually is safe to proceed, though not too abruptly, to the examination.* If there has been a separate interview with the parents, or if for any reason the interview is not conducted in the examining room, some questions should be asked again about the child's current behavior in order to establish the necessary rapport. Thus, an interview also is used as a preparatory stage for the formal behavioral examination.

ORDER OF THE EXAMINATION

The examination sequences for each of the eight key age zones—4, 16, 28, 40 and 52 weeks, 18, 24 and 36 months—are listed on the corresponding developmental schedules in Chapter 3. The sequences are graduated but flexible; no sequence differs drastically from the adjacent ones. The new behavior situations which appear progressively at each age are indicated by italics. The objective is *to learn the general progression of the sequences from age to age,* and how to present the different examination objects, and then observe the responses they evoke. Often it will help in understanding the meaning of a given pattern if similar behavior at adjacent ages is surveyed. Details for conducting the examination procedures themselves are outlined in Chapter 4.

The sequences for 4 and 16 weeks begin with supine situations. The ones for 28, 40 and 52 weeks assume a child who can sit, supported or unsupported. Those for 18, 24 and 36 months assume an ambulatory (locomotor) child who can be seated in front of a small table. To choose the proper sequence for a particular child, determine first the category in which the child fits best. If there are no contraindications, select the sequence nearest to his chronologic age. If obvious deviations, defects, or retardations have been noted, make due allowances. Having selected one sequence, do not fail to shift to a more advanced or a lower one if the child's performance so demands. Adjacent sequences are so closely related that shifts generally do not entail any serious readjustments. However, the standard order of the situations within each sequence should be maintained as far as possible.

The chief point is that the child's demonstrated abilities and interests should determine the specific situations that are used. Your aim is to ascertain the maximum levels of abilities, so it is desirable to stretch adjustment to this maximum. For example, you may be examining a 44-week-old infant on the 40-week sequence; he has given such an excellent performance with the pellet beside the bottle that you might wish to see if he will insert it in the bottle. You may even shift entirely to the 52-week sequence.

Conversely, do not hesitate to start at or shift to a lower sequence. Many unsuccessful examinations, particularly with deviant children, are unsuccessful because the examiner learns during the interview that there are fragments of behavior at, or close to, the child's chronologic age. Therefore, she assumes that the child's developmental age is in the normal range. As a consequence, she remains within this age range in her presentations and obtains meaningless, chaotic behavior which she then diagnoses as psychotic. By dropping abruptly, or gradually, to a much lower age range, she secures behavior revealing of the child's true capacity; those patterns necessary for making a more definitive diagnosis then can be explored.

The examination of a child with motor disabilities always presents practical problems and requires infinite patience. It demands ingenuity in adapting the situations to fit the child, and alertness to the use of substitutive patterns of behavior. It involves the provision of accessory postural aids for successful performance—holding the head firmly supported, lifting the arm to place the hands in a favorable position for prehension, providing adequate sitting support, and even presenting the tabletop situations on the crib platform while the child is in a reclining position, cradling the head of a very young infant in the examiner's hand to inhibit the tonic-neck-reflex and permit head rotation. The objective is to differentiate as precisely as possible motor disability from intellectual defect. Rest periods during which the child is permitted to lie back often permit a renewed attack on the examination with revived zeal and interest.

There is a rationale to the order of presentation within each sequence. Cubes are used at or near the beginning of most of the sequences because the cubes have universal ingratiating appeal. The seriated cube presentations build up an anticipation in an infant which projects itself into ensuing situations. He soon expects you to give him something new to do. This expectation, properly guided and satisfied, imparts flow and dynamic progression to the examination. In general, postural tests are deferred to the end to reduce any possible disturbing effect and to give the child more free play in the examining crib or on the floor.

Since the examination in its entirety is a single unit, the transitions between situations are as important as the situations *per se;* they are neither to be overlooked nor regarded as impediments. It is relatively simple to make a smooth transition from the interview to the formal examination situation. The ambulatory child already has been seated at the examining table during the interview. In the case of an infant, the mother has removed his shoes and stockings during the interview; the remainder of the disrobing is best left until the postural tests are undertaken, unless the clothes interfere with performance prior to this time. The mother places the infant in the proper examining position, and the examiner remains initially at a proper distance. Once an adaptation is made, if she does not spontaneously do so, the mother is asked to remain on the side to allow the examiner full sway. How the mother handles the child throughout, and how the child reacts to her as well as to the examiner, can also provide information which is of diagnostic import. If the child is playing with a toy at the close of the interview, he is permitted to retain the toy, which may be removed as soon as the cubes, for example, are presented. Either he will drop it in response to the new rival toy or you may extract it gently at the moment of cube presentation. By a similar ruse, you may remove the cube before the next object, the pellet, is presented. Some children cling more tightly than others to an object in hand; however, most of them make a prompt adjustment from one object to the next, and once the examination is under way there is little difficulty in accomplishing transitions.

The tempo of the examination should be regulated freely to meet individual requirements. It is impractical and unnecessary to allot a specified amount of time to each of the behavior situations. You will learn empirically how soon a child is ready for the next situation. Sometimes, as with the pellet, a few seconds of exploitation may suffice. However, if the infant shows great eagerness and versatility in his exploitation, for example, of the bell, you may permit him to manipulate it for several minutes. The tempo will differ greatly with each child; one may run through the whole series of situations in less than 10 minutes, but another may take twice as long or more. Certain modes or cycles of exploitation also tend to repeat themselves. Such cycles are characteristic patterns of activity which afford a clue to the timing of the examination situations.

With skillful management, a child's interest in the materials will mount as the examination proceeds. No situation should be allowed to drag or exhaust itself. The examination should not be interrupted to make recordings. One situation should shift into the next with a smooth swing. If necessary, the recommended order may be altered to suit child or exigency. That tempo is best which stimulates, builds up, and sustains the child's interest.

There is one final procedural point applicable to the examination of an infant: the examiner should learn to talk about what the infant is doing as it occurs. This serves several purposes. One is to sharpen the examiner's ability to observe behavior and recall it more completely for subsequent recording. Second, a quietly dictated commentary may actually enhance an infant's performance by eliminating the void of silence.

RECORDING AND DIAGNOSTIC REVIEW

A detailed record of behavior observed during the examination must be added to the historic information obtained. The examiner's commentary during the examination of an infant supplies especially valuable data in complicated cases requiring long supervision. When audio- or videotape recording is available, observations can be captured at the very time they are being made for immediate postexamination review. If no electronic equipment is available, the dictation may be recorded by a stenographer. Since comments by the examiner may interfere with an older child, the stenographic assistant also can be trained to observe and write out a complete account of the child's behavior. Ideally, the assistant should be seated in an inconspicuous corner of the room where no distraction to the examination is offered. Still better is stationing the stenographer behind a one-way screen, described in Appendix C-4 of *Developmental Diagnosis*,[6] which can be installed easily in any office. A final alternative is to recall and jot down pertinent comments immediately after the examination. It is unwise for the examiner to attempt to write any observations during the course of the examination, lest the flow of the child's behavior be interrupted.

A minimal record, which may be adequate for children without abnormalities, consists of plus and minus signs entered on the developmental schedules. In all other instances, a record should be made of the qualitative aspects of behavior and of neuromotor abnormalities described in Chapter 5. Suffice it to say that the plus and minus signs do not automatically deliver a diagnosis. Here, as in all diagnosis, clinical judgment always must be brought to bear. Through experience and study, the examiner should have a fairly well-defined mental image of the normal behavior characteristics of a representative child at any given key age. He also has an image of the behavior characteristics he has just witnessed. He then can match the witnessed behavioral picture against the normal image for the child as a whole, and separately for each of the five fields of behavior. Controlled objectively by the stages embodied in the developmental schedules, such critical comparison permits determination of developmental age.

A thorough knowledge of normal central nervous system function is the basis on which detection of abnormality rests. Familiarity with changes in behavior resulting from localized or generalized dysfunction, as well as an intensive knowledge of the various neuropsychiatric clinical entities, are absolutely essential for more definitive diagnosis and treatment. After reference to the behavioral pictures of various clinical conditions in Chapter 5 and in Part II of *Developmental Diagnosis,* the examiner will discover how the behavior of atypical and defective children deviates from the normal. She will recognize deviations as signs of maldevelopment and will be able to arrive at differential and descriptive diagnoses. She will have a clearer understanding of the more detailed directions for recording and evaluating behavior which are found in Chapter 6.

DISCUSSION OF THE FINDINGS AND RECOMMENDATIONS

Immediately following the recording and diagnostic review of the examination, either by the examiner alone or with students or other personnel who have been involved in the evaluation process, a discussion should be held with the parents. The manner in which the diagnosis is made and imparted to the parents is fundamental to successful guidance, and there are certain principles which should be followed. First, if the parents are to be satisfied with the diagnosis and prognosis given them and receptive to the necessary plans for management, they must know the basis on which the diagnosis is being made. The diagnostic process is thus an integral part of the treatment. Observation of the examination is the way in which the parents best can understand the basis for the diagnosis. It also clarifies their feelings and systematizes their own observations, permits them to see behavior and symptoms which will be important in management, and allows the physician to observe interactions between the child and the parents.

During the postexamination discussion, physician and parents should be seated comfortably and any impression of haste eliminated. If a trial of treatment or further tests are indicated before coming to firm conclusions about prognosis, preliminary findings and the reasons for further steps should be explained. If the physician will take 15 or 20 minutes to cover certain points in a structured fashion, he will find that he usually has answered most of the parents' questions, even though he then may have to go over some points several times. A more detailed discussion of the content of such a conference can be found in Chapter 18 of *Developmental Diagnosis*.

THE WRITTEN REPORT

All the information gathered forms the basis for a written report to the referring physician or agency and for inclusion in the child's record and hospital chart. The purposes of such a report are to clarify in the examiner's mind what he has observed, to give the data on which he is basing his diagnosis, prognosis and recommendations for management, and to transmit this information in a clear and understandable way to others. Certain basic information is included for all patients, but the report should be geared toward specific description of the distinctive abilities and disabilities of the child under consideration. A general outline and illustrative specimen for this report are detailed in Chapter 6.

3
The Revised Developmental Stages

In the preface to this volume we have set forth some of our reasons for why developmental rates have changed. To paraphrase them would be difficult, to repeat them gratuitous. We urge the users of this volume to read them there.

As was true for the original developmental schedules, the derivation of these schedules differs from procedures used in establishing psychometric test norms. Children with evidence of central nervous system dysfunction are excluded. This is the approach used in the establishment of "normal" values in any area of medicine; individuals with disease are excluded. As has been stated already, the term *normal* is, with few exceptions, used in its connotation of *healthy*.

Rather than continuing to use the word "he" generically, and debating how to handle the question of gender, we have alternated the masculine and feminine pronouns for child and examiner alike. The shifts should not prove too jarring.

While the following descriptions of behavior may read rigidly or dogmatically, all should be interpreted as meaning the usual or average behavior. A further word of caution is necessary regarding the descriptions. After the age of 15 or 18 months they apply largely to children raised in middle- and upper-class environments. Behaviors differing from those described are not necessarily indications of developmental defects; rather they may signify differing parental or social mores. Those examination items most socially determined may be biased in favor of white middle-class populations. These social allusions are far from academic; they concern developmental diagnosis. The developmental diagnostician must distinguish the effects of brain damage or impairment, of social differences in rearing, and of social and psychologic damage. He also must prescribe remediation when clinical abnormality is present. Decisions of such importance require careful consideration of individual and sociocultural variation.

To grasp the characteristics of child development, we must think in terms of behavior patterns, maturity stages, and growth trends. The present chapter is organized to facilitate such thinking, by giving a panoramic view of the stream of normal, *that is* healthy, *development in the first 3 years of life. It also supplies a cross-sectional view of that stream at 8 strategic points or key ages: 4, 16, 28, 40 and 52 weeks, 18, 24 and 36 months. These key ages hold a prominent place in developmental diagnosis; they represent the basic stages of maturity to which observed behavior can be referred for appraisal. The discussion for each key age furnishes a guide for defining the behavioral examination, for identifying observed behavior patterns and for interpreting their developmental significance in terms of normal patterns. With these ages well in mind, the student will be oriented, and have the working knowledge of healthy development necessary for an understanding of defects and deviations.*

To examine a child of a specific age, first read the narrative text most appropriate for the child's age and look at the action drawings which accompany it. Next look at the developmental schedules, which list the behavior patterns in abbreviated form, and read the glossary. The glossary defines more precisely the meaning of these necessarily shortened behavior patterns which will be seen in the formal examination. It also indicates the manner in which patterns should be inquired about, particularly the language and personal-social behavior one would not necessarily expect to observe. Finally, review the examination sequence which appears beside the Key Age developmental schedule and read the instructions for each specific situation listed. These specific instructions appear in Chapter 4.

ORGANIZATION OF THE CHAPTER

To emphasize the continuity of development and the essential similarity of examination methods, each key age is treated in the same manner.

Narrative Text. The accompanying text provides a condensed narrative picture of the developmental examination and of typical behavior for each key age. In the text, each examination situation is indicated by the words spelled in CAPITAL LETTERS. *Italics* are used to specify all behavior which appears characteristically for the first time at each key age.

Action Drawings. Action pictures portray the behavior patterns that are diagnostically significant. These behavior patterns are representative and typical; they delineate the kinds of reactions elicited by developmental examination.

Developmental Schedule. The developmental schedule codifies behavior patterns for diagnostic application. It is especially advantageous to consider a key age in relation to the 2 age levels immediately adjacent—the next younger and older. Accordingly, for the 1st year of life each schedule lists the behavior characteristics of the key age and its 2 adjacent ages in 3 vertical columns. The key age occupies the central position. From 15–36 months, 2 ages are placed on facing pages. Horizontally, the behavior characteristics are grouped by the five major behavioral fields—adaptive, gross motor, fine motor, language, and personal-social. This arrangement permits ready cross-comparison in terms of kinds of behavior as well as levels of maturity.

The behavior patterns arrayed in a single age column should not be regarded as isolated "test" items. They are closely correlated and must be considered a compact organic characterization of the behavior typical for that age. These behavior patterns are the diagnostic criteria for evaluating observed behavior. Two kinds of patterns appear: (1) *permanent patterns* which come to stay or augment, and (2) *temporary patterns* which give way or transform into different and more advanced patterns at later ages. A child builds a tower of 2 cubes at 56 weeks; of 3 at 15 months. This is clearly a permanent type of behavior pattern. An infant of 12 weeks sits supported with bobbing head, and one of 16 weeks sits with head steady. Steadiness supersedes the temporary pattern of bobbing and is permanent. A temporary pattern is indicated on the developmental schedules by an asterisk, followed by the age at which it is replaced by a more mature pattern of the same nature.

On each of the developmental schedules, certain items in the history columns have been blocked out, indicating that these patterns are so precisely defined that the behavior must be observed by the examiner.

Glossary of Behavior Patterns. The items which appear on the schedules are for the most part self-explanatory. However, they are worded briefly. A glossary is necessary to clarify abbreviations of statement and to specify details. It is placed in the text rather than in a separate appendix to facilitate understanding of the precise meaning of each behavior pattern. Clarification will be enhanced further by reading the descriptions at adjacent age levels.

Examination Sequence. For each key age, the narrative text is summarized by a tabulation of the order in which the examination situations are carried out. The situation numbers refer to the detailed description of the examination procedures found in Chapter 4. Reference also should be made to Chapter 2, where the general approach to the evaluation is discussed.

The examination procedures in Chapter 4 are arranged according to the general character of the situations, with the ages to which each applies grouped within them. They give specific instructions for the manner in which the situation is to be administered.

The narrative test, the glossary, and the examination procedures each provide additional clarification for the others and should be read as a single unit.

The key ages correspond to 3 developmental periods, or maturity zones, which indicate the usual starting position for the examination.

Key Ages	*Maturity Zones*
4 weeks	Supine (crib)
16 weeks	
28 weeks	Sitting (crib)
40 weeks	
52 weeks	
18 months	Locomotor (child's table and chair)
24 months	
36 months	

Three definitions will obviate repetition in the ensuing material:
Supine: lying face up.
Prone: lying face down.
Sitting: implies with support until the age of 36 weeks.

The dangling ring and rattle are presented with the infant in the supine position. The bird call and bell-ring (to elicit a response to sound) are presented when the infant is supine at 4–24 weeks, sitting from 28–56 weeks, and opportunistically with older children when hearing loss is suspected. All other objects are presented with the child in the sitting position.

In determining the age of an infant or child at the time of examination, the following procedures should be used:

Through 59 weeks: take the midpoint of the week; *e.g.*, 40 weeks includes the period from 39 weeks and 4 days through 40 weeks and 3 days.

14 months and over: use whole and half-month age intervals and include 8 days on either side of the midpoint; *e.g.*, 18 months includes the period from 17 months and 24 days through 18 months and 8 days; 18.5 months covers the period from 18 months and 9 days through 18 months and 23 days.

In the case of premature birth, the *chronologic age must be corrected* by the amount of prematurity (see Chapter 12 of *Developmental Diagnosis*).

4 WEEKS OR LESS

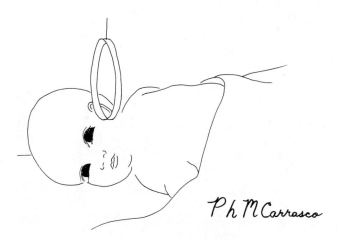

Follows to midline, not beyond

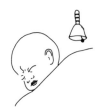

Facial response

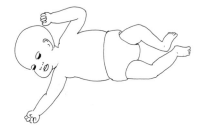

Tonic-neck-reflex predominates, hands fisted

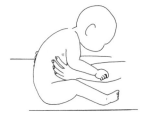

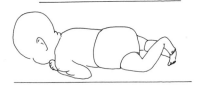

Barely lifts head, hips high

Head sags, back rounded

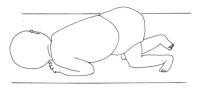

Head rotates, crawling movements

The most opportune time to examine the 4-week-old infant is when he is neither drowsy nor hungry. Even so, his *expression* wears a remote, *impassive* detachment. His spontaneous *regard* is *staring* and *indirect,* and remains so when he is placed on his back in SUPINE for observation. He lies in the *tonic-neck-reflex (t-n-r) position.* His *head* is *turned* far *to the side,* with the arm and leg on that side extended; the other arm is flexed close to the shoulder or occiput, and that leg also is flexed. His *hands* are tightly *fisted;* sometimes one goes to the mouth. When active he makes more or less symmetric windmill movements, extending one or both arms sharply. He flexes and extends the legs, lifting them an inch or two.

He disregards the DANGLING RING in the midplane, but when it is brought into his *line of vision* he *regards* it. When it is moved slowly toward the midplane again he *follows* it with combined eye and some head movements *to the midline,* but *not beyond,* and then returns his head to its preferred side position.

The RATTLE also is disregarded in the midplane and only momentarily in the *line of vision.* When the handle of the rattle is touched to the fisted fingers, he *clenches* his *fist on contact,* and his fingers must be pried open to receive the rattle. He *retains it briefly.*

The examiner faces the infant, bends over and smiles and talks in SOCIAL STIMULATION. The baby responds by *immobilizing* his *activity,* and he *regards the examiner's face.*

When the examiner activates the BIRD CALL softly by each ear in turn the infant *attends, reducing his activity;* his eyes may widen or his brows furrow in a *facial response.* If there is no response to this soft sound, a BELL is RUNG near each ear.

By gentle maneuvers the examiner institutes a few postural tests to determine muscular tonicity and motor response. By holding the infant's hands, a tentative pull toward the perpendicular sitting position is exerted. PULL-TO-SITTING is not completed if, as is usual at this age, the *head* falls back with *complete* or marked *lag.*

When held in the SUPPORTED SITTING position, the baby's *head sags* forward on his chest, although he may lift it momentarily. His *back* is evenly *rounded.*

In SUPPORTED STANDING, the examiner's hands around the chest below the armpits, the legs extend briefly and the toes flex, but resistance to the table surface is slight or wanting.

The infant then is held in VENTRAL SUSPENSION above the crib surface. *Head* and *legs* droop, showing *no postural compensation.* He is lowered to the crib PRONE, and just as he is placed down he *rotates his head* so that he rests on his cheek. His arms are flexed close to his head, and the legs are in a kneeling position with his *hips high.* He extends and draws up his legs in *crawling movements.* The baby *barely lifts his head* just clear of the crib surface and then returns it to the side.

Vocalizations are confined to *small throaty sounds.* The mother reports that the infant startles easily to sudden sounds or movements, sometimes without apparent external cause, and that he requires *2 feedings* during the *night* after the early evening feeding.

EXAMINATION SEQUENCE
Supine (Crib)

0–4–8 Weeks	Situation No.*
Supine	1
Dangling Ring	2
Rattle	3
Social Stimulation	4
Bird Call, Bell-Ring	5
Pull-to-Sitting	6
Sitting Supported	62
Standing Supported	63
Ventral Suspension	64
Prone	65

*Situation number identifies the examination situation described in Chapter 4, Examination Procedures.

H = History
O = Observation
(*) = Pattern replaced by more mature one at later age.

KEY AGE: 4 Weeks Or Less

H	O	
		ADAPTIVE
		Dangling Ring, Rattle: regards, line of vision only (*8w)
		Dangling Ring, Rattle: follows to midline, not beyond (*8w)
		Rattle: retains briefly (*16w)
		Bird Call, Bell-Ring: attends, reduces activity (*24w)
		Bird Call, Bell-Ring: facial response (*24w)
		GROSS MOTOR
		Supine: side position head predominates (*12w)
		Supine: tonic-neck-reflex (t-n-r) position predominates (*12w)
		Pull-to-Sit: complete head lag (*20w)
		Sit: head sags (*8w)
		Sit: back rounded (*16w)
		Ventral Suspension: no head or leg compensation (*8w)
		Prone Placement: head rotates (*12w)
		Prone: barely lifts head (*8w)
		Prone: hips high (*8w)
		Prone: crawling movements (*8w)
		FINE MOTOR
		Dangling Ring, Rattle: hand clenches on contact (*16w)
		Supine: hands fisted (*12w)
		LANGUAGE
		Expression: impassive face (*8w)
		Expression: indirect regard (*8w)
		Vocalization: small throaty noises (*8w)
		PERSONAL-SOCIAL
		Supine: stares indefinitely (*8w)
		Social: regards examiner, reduces activity (*8w)
		Feeding: 2 night feedings (*8w)

H	O	8 Weeks
		ADAPTIVE
		Dangling Ring, Rattle: delayed midline regard (*12w)
		Dangling Ring: follows past midline (*16w)
		Dangling Ring: follows vertically
		GROSS MOTOR
		Supine: head mid-position seen (*12w)
		Supine: symmetric postures seen (*12w)
		Sit: head bobbingly erect (*12w)
		Ventral Suspension: head compensates, not legs (*16w)
		Prone: head to 45° recurrently (*12w)
		Prone: hips low, frog position (*16w)
		FINE MOTOR
		Dangling Ring: retains
		LANGUAGE
		Expression: alert face
		Expression: direct regard
		Vocalization: "talks back"
		Vocalization: single vowel sounds (*28w)
		Vocalization: coos (*28w)
		PERSONAL-SOCIAL
		Supine: regards examiner recurrently (*12w)
		Social: follows moving person
		Social: smiles responsively
		Feeding: 1 night feeding ("———)

A complete set of 8 developmental schedules in standard 8½- by 11-inch size is available from the authors. As described on page 19, there are 3 ages per page for the 4- to 56-week age range, and 2 per page for 15 to 36 months.

GLOSSARY

4 Weeks or Less

ADAPTIVE

Dangling Ring, Rattle: regards, line of vision only. Object perceived only when brought into direct line of vision at favorable focal distance (about 12 inches).

Dangling Ring, Rattle: follows to midline, not beyond. Infant follows with eyes, with or without turning head, definitely fixating upon object. Does not merely make random movements which examiner then follows.

Rattle: retains briefly. When fingers opened by examiner and rattle placed, it is held against crib surface passively and momentarily before it drops.

Bird Call, Bell-Ring: attends, reduces activity. Response may be very brief; infant may inhibit respiration momentarily. Differentiate definite evidence of listening from reflex blink response.

Bird Call, Bell-Ring: facial response. Eye widening, frown, grimace, etc., accompany inhibition of activity.

GROSS MOTOR

Supine: side position head predominates. Head held predominantly turned to side. May be preference for one side, or sides may alternate.

Supine: tonic-neck-reflex (t-n-r) position predominates. Head turned to side, arm and leg extended on same side; opposite arm and leg flexed—the fencing position. Position observed spontaneously, not elicited, but infant must be awake and lying on a surface which is firm and large enough not to restrict body movements.

Pull-to-Sitting: complete head lag. As infant is pulled toward sitting by holding hands, head sags backwards. Pull cannot be completed without support to head.

Sitting: head sags. When held supported in sitting position, chin rests on chest.

Sitting: back rounded. When held in sitting position infant's back resembles C-curve.

Ventral Suspension: no head or leg compensation. When held face down with examiner's hands on chest below armpits, infant forms an inverted U.

Prone Placement: head rotates. Placed face down, head turns to side and infant rests on cheek.

Prone: barely lifts head. Lifts head so face barely clears crib surface, or so chin is about one inch above surface.

Prone: hips high. Hips raised in air. Infant's knees usually flexed and legs tucked up underneath.

Prone: crawling movements. Legs only; arms inactive and tucked under chest.

FINE MOTOR

Dangling Ring, Rattle: hand clenches on contact. Fisted hand fists more tightly when touched by ring or rattle handle; hand may open eventually.

Supine: hands fisted. When infant is awake, hands primarily fisted, thumb resting outside clenched fingers.

LANGUAGE

Expression: impassive face. For most of examination period.

Expression: indirect regard. Definite fixation not sustained.

Vocalization: small throaty noises. Soft unformed sounds.

PERSONAL-SOCIAL

Supine: stares indefinitely. Definite fixation not sustained.

Social: regards examiner, reduces activity. In response to examiner's nodding and talking. Touching infant's face not included in social stimulation.

Feeding: 2 night feedings. After early evening (approximately 6 P.M.) feeding.

8 Weeks

ADAPTIVE

Dangling Ring, Rattle: delayed midline regard. When ring or rattle is brought up from level of feet to above chest, infant eventually turns head, catches sight of and fixates upon object, or upon examiner's hand holding it.

Dangling Ring: follows past midline. Follows ring or examiner's hand; some head rotation necessary. Does not follow rattle.

Dangling Ring: follows vertically. Follows upward and downward motion when ring moved vertically slowly. Eye coordination may not be smooth. Does not follow rattle.

GROSS MOTOR

Supine: head mid-position seen. Chin and nose in line with median line of trunk; tonic-neck-reflex (t-n-r) less stereotyped and less persistent.

Supine: symmetric postures seen. Arms and legs symmetrically disposed. Posture not predominant, but observed.

Sitting: head bobbingly erect. In supported sitting position, head sags forward with chin on or near chest, but lifts to erect position recurrently.

Ventral Suspension: head compensates, not legs. Head held in line with trunk as infant lowered in prone position with examiner's hands on chest below armpits. Legs still droop.

Prone: head to 45° recurrently. Chin lifts 2 to 3 inches above crib surface. Head falls down again, without control of movement.

Prone: hips low, frog position. Hips no longer flexed, thighs rest on crib surface. Hips abducted, knees usally remaining flexed.

FINE MOTOR

Dangling Ring: retains. Placed ring stays off crib surface for brief period, even though hand opens and closes on it. Top-heavy rattle falls.

LANGUAGE

Expression: alert face. Watchful, wide-awake expression.

Expression: direct regard. Visual attention focused for most of examination.

Vocalization: "talks back." Infant vocalizes in some manner, in response to social stimulation. (See 4 weeks, *Social.*)

Vocalization: single vowel sounds. Ah, eh, uh.

Vocalization: coos. Sustained single vowel sounds, "aaah . . . ooo . . . ," like murmuring of pigeon.

PERSONAL-SOCIAL

Supine: regards examiner recurrently. Looks at examiner spontaneously and selectively but not for long periods.

Social: follows moving person. Follows person who crosses line of vision. Eye movements may not be smooth but definite tracking elicited.

Social: smiles responsively. Facial brightening or smiling in response to examiner's nodding head and talking. (See 4 weeks, *Social.*)

Feeding: 1 night feeding. After early evening (approximately 6 P.M.) feeding.

16 WEEKS

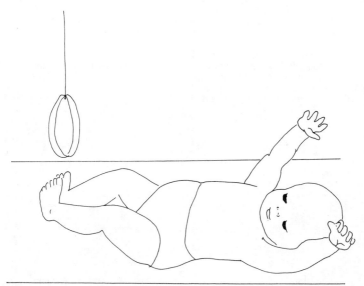

PhMC

Regards immediately, arms activate

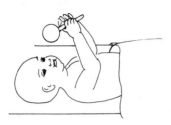

Regards in hand

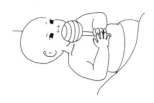

To mouth, free hand fingers

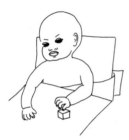

Contacts

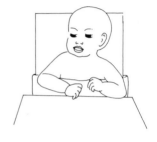

Delayed recurrent regard

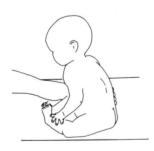

Head set forward, steady

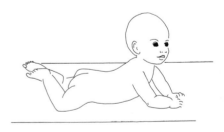

Head 90° sustainedly, legs extended

The 16-week-old baby inspects persons and surroundings with much more alertness than the 4-week-old. This is due in part to the marked advance in eye and head control. When she is placed on her back in SUPINE, the midposition of the head and symmetric postures are well established. Her *hands engage* with mutual fingering near her face or over her chest, or are flung out in lateral extension at shoulder level. Fingers are extended or only slightly flexed. She looks at the examiner and *initiates a social smile*. She fixates readily on any object which moves into her visual field.

She *regards immediately* the DANGLING RING held over her feet in the midplane and *follows the ring* or the examiner's hand holding the string from one side to the other *through an arc of 180°*. Interest in the examiner's face frequently interferes with ring-following at this very social age. When the ring is suspended over her chest, her *arms activate;* when it is placed in her hand, her *hand curls around it actively*. She *regards it*, holds it, *brings it to her mouth*, and *fingers or holds it with her free hand*. Her behavior with the RATTLE is similar, as she is able now to *retain* the top-heavy *rattle* as easily as the ring.

The examiner faces the infant for SOCIAL STIMULATION. The 16-week baby initiates the social approach, smiling in response to the examiner's presence. The examiner then activates the BIRD CALL softly a few inches from each ear in turn. The baby attends to the sound by abating activity. She may blink, frown, smile, or even cry. If there is no response to this soft sound, a hand BELL is RUNG briskly near each ear.

The examiner takes the baby's hands for PULL-TO-SITTING. Her head lags only slightly and she *smiles or vocalizes pleasantly* on attaining the sitting position.

Placed in a supporting chair or held seated at the table, she is interested in toys as well as in the examiner. She holds her *head steady but set forward*. She *fingers and scratches* actively on the tabletop.

When the FIRST CUBE is presented she *regards it immediately, activates her arms* and succeeds in *contacting* the single cube. She *holds one cube placed* in her hands and *regards the* SECOND CUBE as it is brought in. The MASSED CUBES (or a CUP) are more likely to elicit a grasp on contact since they have greater stimulus value than a single cube.

(Text continued p. 37)

	Situation No. *
12–16–20 Weeks	
Supine	1
Dangling Ring	2
Rattle	3
Social Stimulation	4
Bird Call, Bell-Ring	5
Pull-to-Sitting	6
Chair–Tabletop	
Cubes 1, 2, 3	7,8,9
Massed Cubes	11
Cup	16
Pellet	20
Yarn	26
Bell	24
Mirror	32
Sitting Supported	62
Standing Supported	63
Ventral Suspension	64
Prone	65

Italicized items appear for the first time in this sequence.

*Situation number identifies the examination situation described in Chapter 4, Examination Procedures.

H = History
O = Observation
(*) = Pattern replaced by more mature one at later age.

KEY AGE: 16 Weeks

H	O	
		ADAPTIVE
	▨	Dangling Ring, Rattle: regards immediately
		Dangling Ring, Rattle: arms activate (*20w)
		Dangling Ring, Rattle: achieves 180° arc
	▨	Dangling Ring, Rattle: regards in hand
	▨	Dangling Ring, Rattle: to mouth
		Dangling Ring, Rattle: free hand fingers, holds
		Cube, Bell: regards immediately
		Cube, Bell: arms activate (*20w)
		Cube, Bell: contacts (*20w)
		2nd Cube: holds 1 placed, regards 2nd (*28w)
		Yarn: follows 180° in air
		Pellet: delayed recurrent regard (*24w)
		GROSS MOTOR
	▨	Supine: hands engage
		Sit: head set forward, steady (*20w)
		Sit: lumbar curvature only (*24w)
		Ventral Suspension: head, legs compensate
		Prone: head to 90° sustainedly
		Prone: legs extended
		Prone: 1 arm flexed, 1 extended (*20w)
		Prone: rolls to supine
		FINE MOTOR
	▨	Dangling Ring, Rattle: hand curls actively
		Rattle: retains
		Tabletop: fingers, scratches table
		LANGUAGE
		Expressive: breathes heavily, excites (*24w)
		Vocalization: laughs out loud
		Vocalization: squeals
		Vocalization: "talks" to toys or people spontaneously
		PERSONAL-SOCIAL
		Feeding: pats bottle, both hands (*36w)
		Social: smiles, vocalizes, pull-to-sit (*24w)
		Social: spontaneous social smile
		Play: sits propped 10–15 minutes
	▨	Play: pulls clothes over face (*24w)
		Mirror: smiles & vocalizes

H	O	12 Weeks		H	O	20 Weeks
		ADAPTIVE				**ADAPTIVE**
		Dangling Ring, Rattle: prompt midline regard (*16w)				Dangling Ring, Rattle: 2-hand approach (*28w)
		Dangling Ring, Rattle: glances at in hand (*16w)				Dangling Ring, Rattle: grasps by completing distance (*24w)
		Dangling Ring: circular coordination				Rattle: looks after lost rattle
		Rattle: follows past midline (*16w)				Cube: 2-hand approach (*28w)
		Rattle: follows vertically				3rd Cube: holds 2 placed, regards 3rd (*28W)
		Tabletop: regards table or hands				Massed Cubes: grasps 1 on contact (*24w)
		Massed Cubes, Cup: regards immediately				Massed Cubes: exploits 2 cubes
		Massed Cubes, Cup: regards prolongedly				Bell: 2-hand approach and grasp (*28w)
		Massed Cubes, Cup: arms activate (*20w)				Yarn: turns head after fallen yarn
		Yarn: follows across table				
		GROSS MOTOR				**GROSS MOTOR**
		Supine: head mid-position predominates				Supine: lifts legs high in extension
		Supine: symmetric postures predominate				Pull-to-Sit: no head lag
		Sit: head set forward, bobs (*16w)				Sit: head erect, steady
		Stand: small fraction weight briefly (*20w)				Ventral Suspension: arms extend
		Prone Place: head midline sustained				Prone: both elbows extended
		Prone: head to 45° sustainedly				Stand: large fraction weight
		Prone: head to platform with control				Stand: shoulder tone sustained
		Prone: rests on forearms spontaneously				
		FINE MOTOR				**FINE MOTOR**
		Supine: hands open or loosely closed				Cube: precarious grasp (*24w)
		Supine: fingers, scratches (*24w)				
		Dangling Ring, Rattle: holds actively, placed (*16w)				
		Massed Cubes, Cup: contacts (*20w)				
		LANGUAGE				**LANGUAGE**
		Vocalization: chuckles				Vocalization: grunts, growls
		PERSONAL-SOCIAL				**PERSONAL-SOCIAL**
		Supine: regards examiner predominantly (*——)				Dangling Ring, Rattle: mouthes (*28w)
		Feeding: anticipates food on sight				Social: discriminates strangers
		Play: hand regard (*——)				
		Play: hand play, mutual fingering (*24w)				

She follows the examiner's withdrawing hand when the PELLET is presented, regards her own hands, and finally gives the pellet *delayed recurrent regard*.

She *follows the dangled ball* of YARN *180°* as it is moved across in a smooth arc at her eye level.

The BELL also evokes *prompt* and prolonged *regard* and she succeeds in *contacting* it.

The table is removed, the infant taken out of the chair and placed close to a large MIRROR. She *smiles and talks* to her mirror image. When she is turned to face the examiner in a SUPPORTED SITTING position she requires firm support, but her back shows only a *lumbar curvature*.

The infant then is held in the STANDING position SUPPORTED around the chest below the armpits. She sustains a moderate fraction of weight for a short period.

When held in VENTRAL SUSPENSION above the crib she keeps her *head and legs in good alignment with her trunk*. As she is placed PRONE in the crib, she maintains the midposition of her head, holding it *sustainedly lifted to a 90° angle*. A toy may be used as a lure to induce head-lifting. Her *legs are extended* and she props on her forearms. Because *one arm is flexed*, the *other* more *extended*, and the head position high, her prone equilibrium is unstable and she *rolls* involuntarily *to a supine position*.

In her interest in the examination toys she may *strain, breathe fast*, purse her lips, and show other evidences of excitement. She is reported to *laugh out loud* and *squeal* with high-pitched vocalization. She is a vocal individual now and starts to *"talk" to her toys or other people spontaneously*.

She is reported to *pat her bottle with both hands* and *pull clothes over her face* as her arms move up and down. She *sits propped* erect with pillows in the corner of a sofa or crib *for 10–15 minutes*.

12 Weeks

ADAPTIVE

Dangling Ring, Rattle: prompt midline regard. When ring or rattle reaches chest level, infant regards object in midline, turning head from partly side position to do so if necessary.

Dangling Ring, Rattle: glances at in hand. Be certain infant looks at placed rattle or ring rather than at some distant point beyond it. Infant frequently does not lift object from crib in this situation.

Dangling Ring: circular coordination. Infant follows dangling ring in full circle; eye movements may be jerky rather than smoothly coordinated.

Rattle: follows past midline. As rattle moves past midline infant follows with eyes; some head turning necessary. Be certain infant is fixating upon rattle, not merely making random movements which examiner then follows.

Rattle: follows vertically. Follows upward and downward motion when rattle moved vertically slowly. Eye coordination may not be smooth.

Tabletop: regards table or hands. Spontaneously regards table surface or own hands on table, in absence of object.

Massed Cubes, Cup: regards immediately. When large object tapped at far edge of tabletop, infant gives immediate definite regard.

Massed Cubes, Cup: regards prolongedly. After large object brought within reach, infant gives definite sustained regard.

Massed Cubes, Cup: arms activate. During regard for large object. (See 16 weeks.)

Yarn: follows across table. As yarn moves slowly across tabletop infant follows completely from one side to other though not necessarily in smooth continuous arc.

GROSS MOTOR

Supine: head mid-position predominates. Chin and nose held primarily in line with median line of trunk, and head rotates freely from side to side.

Supine: symmetric postures predominate. Both arms held simultaneously either abducted or with hands together in midline; both legs either extended or flexed.

Sitting: head set forward, bobs. In supported sitting position, head primarily erect but set forward at angle to trunk. It bobs forward towards chest recurrently, even when body is immobile.

Standing: small fraction of weight briefly. Infant held by examiner's hands on chest below armpits; when examiner relaxes support, infant maintains erect position for moment before flexing at hips and knees.

Prone Placement: head midline sustained. When placed face down infant maintains head in midline rather than turning it to side.

Prone: head to 45° sustainedly. Infant maintains chin 2 to 3 inches above crib surface.

Prone: head to platform with control. Infant puts head down rather than letting it fall forward.

Prone: rests on forearms spontaneously. Placed in prone position, infant maintains forearms clear of chest rather than tucked up underneath. Both elbows flexed, weight on elbows and forearms.

FINE MOTOR

Supine: hands open or loosely closed. Hands no longer need to be pried open; ring or rattle placed with ease.

Supine: fingers, scratches. Own body, hair or dress, or may clutch at examiner's clothes on contact.

Dangling Ring, Rattle: holds actively, placed. Active grasp indicated either by lifting of object from crib surface or by whitening of knuckle joints.

Massed Cubes, Cup: contacts. During regard for large object, one or both hands brought against it.

LANGUAGE

Vocalization: chuckles. Just short of true laughter.

PERSONAL-SOCIAL

Supine: regards examiner predominantly. In preference to objects presented.

Feeding: anticipates food on sight. Infant becomes excited and eager when sees bottle or breast, before it is touched to lips.

Play: hand regard. In spontaneous play, infant brings one or both hands before face for regard.

Play: hand play, mutual fingering. Hands finger each other as infant brings them together in spontaneous play.

16 Weeks

Dangling Ring, Rattle: regards immediately. Infant sees object as soon as it is brought over feet.

Dangling Ring, Rattle: arms activate. During regard for object, infant's arms become active, though not necessarily brought near object. Activity may be confined to tremulous poising.

Dangling Ring, Rattle: achieves 180° arc. Eyes and head follow object or examiner's hand to crib surface to each side, but not necessarily in smooth arc.

Dangling Ring, Rattle: regards in hand. Sustained regard of placed object; usually lifts off crib surface to look at it.

Dangling Ring, Rattle: to mouth. Object, not infant's hand, contacts mouth, even though awkwardly and recurrently.

Dangling Ring, Rattle: free hand fingers, holds. Hand approaches object and touches it. Sometimes holds with both hands at same time.

Cube, Bell: regards immediately. As soon as small object is tapped at far edge of table top, infant definitely looks at it.

Cube, Bell: arms activate. Same description as supine (above), but seen in sitting position, and for small object.

Cube, Bell: contacts. During regard for small object, one or both hands brought against it.

2nd Cube: holds 1st placed, regards 2nd. After 1st cube placed in hand, infant maintains contact with it and definitely looks at 2nd as it is brought in from far edge of tabletop.

Yarn: follows 180° in air. As yarn moves in line of vision above surface of tabletop, infant follows from one side to the other.

Pellet: delayed recurrent regard. Any regard that is definite. Examiner may point to pellet to attract attention to it, move it about, etc.; infant tends to follow examiner's withdrawing hand, even if it is removed slowly.

Supine: hands engage. Hands come together spontaneously over chest, and fingers touch *when infant is lying down* on a hard flat surface. Cradling an infant so that head is in midline may force hands together.

Sitting: head set forward, steady. In supported sitting position, head held steady but thrust forward at an angle to body; may bob forward occasionally when arms or trunk move or head turns, but not when infant is immobile.

Sitting: lumbar curvature only. Only lower portion of spine shows rounding; upper trunk is straight in supported sitting position.

Ventral Suspension: head and legs compensate. When held face down with examiner's hands on chest below armpits, head and legs held in line with body.

Prone: head to 90° sustainedly. Infant raises head and looks straight ahead; holds it there with control.

Prone: legs extended. Anterior aspect of thighs rests on crib surface; hips not abducted although knees may flex.

Prone: one arm flexed, one extended. When head is held at 90° angle, infant shows tendency to roll passively over extended arm.

Prone: rolls to supine. Infant turns passively from abdomen to back.

FINE MOTOR

Dangling Ring, Rattle: hand curls actively. As object is touched to infant's hand, hand opens actively to grasp object and closes on it; infant retains it for more than brief period.

Rattle: retains. After being grasped, rattle remains in hand for about 1 minute as infant exploits it. Hands no longer open and close automatically; if they do, top-heavy rattle falls.

Tabletop: fingers, scratches table. Fingers scratch actively, whether or not stimulus object is present.

LANGUAGE

Expressive: breathes heavily, excites. Strains during regard for object.

Vocalization: laughs out loud. Spontaneously, or in response to social stimulation; not to tickling or roughhouse.

Vocalization: squeals. Infant modulates pitch of airstream to high sound resembling squealing pig.

Vocalization: "talks" to toys or people spontaneously. Infant initiates social play by smiling and vocalizing.

PERSONAL-SOCIAL

Feeding: pats bottle, both hands. Infant puts both hands on bottle or breast, as if to hold it.

Social: smiles, vocalizes, pulled-to-sitting. A pleasurable response, apparently in response to translocation and new posture; sometimes almost squeals with delight. Crying not acceptable.

Social: spontaneous social smile. Infant initiates social play by beaming smile in response to examiner's presence, before social advances are made.

Play: sits propped 10–15 minutes. Maintains upright position when placed in corner of sofa or crib with aid of pillows; half-reclining in infant carrier of some type not acceptable.

Play: pulls clothes over face. As arms move up and down, already clutched clothes or blanket comes up over infant's face.

Mirror: smiles and vocalizes. Infant gives definite regard to mirror image, smiles and "talks" to it. Crying not equated with vocalizing.

20 Weeks

ADAPTIVE

Dangling Ring, Rattle: 2-hand approach. In supine position, both hands brought slowly toward presented object with control.

Dangling Ring, Rattle: grasps by completing distance. When object brought within an inch of palmar side of hand, approach completed and object grasped.

Rattle: looks after lost rattle. If rattle drops within sight on crib (or examiner removes it while infant is regarding rattle and places it), head turns to look for it.

Cube: 2-hand approach. In supported sitting position, both hands brought slowly toward presented object with control.

Third Cube: holds 2 placed, regards 3rd. Infant maintains contact with first 2 cubes which have been placed, looks at 3rd cube as it is presented and follows as it is brought in from far edge of tabletop.

Massed Cubes: grasps 1 on contact. Hand falls upon or contacts cubes, with regardful approach or regard after contact, and cube then grasped.

Massed Cubes: exploits 2 cubes. During entire situation infant manages to contact or grasp 2 cubes.

Bell: 2-hand approach and grasp. Approach and grasp synthesized into single coordinated movement in direct response to visual stimulus of bell.

Yarn: turns head after fallen yarn. As yarn moves slowly across tabletop and drops off edge, infant definitely turns head towards side where yarn has disappeared.

GROSS MOTOR

Supine: lifts legs high in extension. Infant lifts legs high enough to see feet.

Pull-to-Sitting: no head lag. Head maintained in line with trunk throughout.

Sitting: head erect, steady. In supported sitting position, head maintained in line with trunk; turns and moves freely at all times without bobbing.

Ventral Suspension: arms extend. When infant is held face down with examiner's hands on chest below armpits and is lowered to platform, arms extend as if in protective motion.

Prone: both elbows extended. Arms held forward as props, resting weight on hands, with entire chest off crib and elbows straight.

Standing: large fraction of weight. When examiner holds infant by placing hands on chest below armpits, hips extend and knees usually flex slightly as infant maintains most of weight.

Standing: shoulder tone sustained. As examiner places hands in infant's armpits and lifts, shoulder tone sustained and infant does not "slide through" examiner's hands.

FINE MOTOR

Precarious grasp

Cube: precarious grasp. Cube held momentarily between fingers and palm, usually at ulnar side, when placed in hand, or on spontaneous grasp. Must lift cube off tabletop, not merely maintain contact.

LANGUAGE

Vocalization: grunts and growls. Modifies airstream with low-pitched sounds, at times other than when having bowel movement.

PERSONAL-SOCIAL

Dangling Ring, Rattle: mouths. Definite licking and mouthing movements when object brought to mouth. (See 28 weeks.)

Social: discriminates strangers. Knows difference between strangers and family. Not necessarily fearful; may simply sober and not accept strangers as quickly as familiars.

28 WEEKS

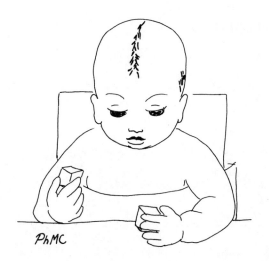

Grasps 1st, grasps 2nd

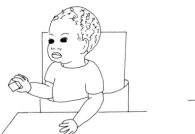

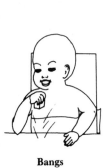

1-hand approach & grasp

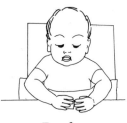

Transfers

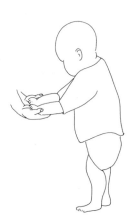

Bangs

Stands, hands held

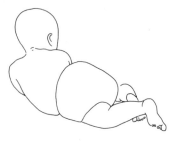

Pivots

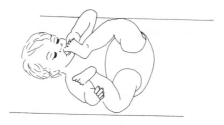

Feet to mouth

The 28-week-old infant sits in the supporting chair with his trunk erect and steady. The introductory toy is removed after a brief period, and the examiner presents the FIRST of three CUBES. The baby *reaches with one hand*, seizes the first cube immediately with a *radial palmar grasp* and carries it to his mouth. While retaining the first cube, *he grasps the* SECOND CUBE and *retains these two more than momentarily*. He *holds these two cubes* which he has grasped *as the* THIRD CUBE *is presented*, but eventually drops one or both when the third comes within reach. He *bangs*, mouthes, *transfers*, drops, and resecures cubes.

He approaches the MASSED CUBES with both hands, secures two cubes and *retains both of them more than momentarily*. When the CUP is added after the infant has grasped a cube, he *retains the cube and grasps the cup*.

He may follow the examiner's withdrawing hand as the PELLET is presented, but then returns to give it intent regard, *rake at it with the radial digits*, or attempt some thumb opposition with an *unsuccessful inferior scissors grasp*. He exploits the BOTTLE WITH THE PELLET INSIDE and may notice the pellet if it falls on to the tabletop.

He turns his head to look down for the fallen YARN which the examiner has pulled across the table and dropped over the edge.

When auditory responses are tested by activation of the BIRD CALL or, if necessary, by RINGING THE BELL opposite each ear in succession, he turns his head correctly and promptly.

He makes an *immediate one-hand approach* to the BELL, taking it by the bowl or junction. He *bangs, bites, and chews* and *transfers* the bell *adeptly, retaining* it without dropping during his exploitation.

The RING-STRING is presented, the string within reach. He has an *inferior scissors grasp* of the string and *secures the ring by the string*, although he does not yet see the connection between them. He manipulates the ring as he does cube and bell.

The table is removed and he is placed in front of the large MIRROR. He reaches for and pats his mirror image. Turned to face the examiner on the crib in a SITTING POSITION, he *sits erect for about one minute* before he either topples over or returns to sitting propped on his hands.

In SUPPORTED STANDING he maintains his trunk erect and steady with his *hands held at shoulder height* just for balance and with his elbows fully extended.

Placed PRONE, he *pivots* in circular translocation by the alternating movements of his arms, usually crossing one over the other. He gets on hands and knees in the *creeping position*. He moves forward by *crawling* flat on his abdomen in an army crawl, or by getting on hands and knees and then falling forward on his abdomen in a *creep-crawl*.

The occasional infant who is not this mature is placed SUPINE. He is given the RATTLE immediately, which he shakes and pursues if it drops.

He is turned to face the examiner who engages him with SOCIAL STIMULATION while his auditory responses are tested, if he did not respond to the BIRD CALL or BELL-RING in the sitting position.

As he is PULLED-TO-SITTING, he assists by lifting his head and flexing his elbows as soon as the pull begins.

His reported language includes combined vowel sounds produced with control, such as *ah-ah-ah, oh-oh-oh;* he says *mum-mum-mum* when he cries. He also makes *single consonants* such as *da, ba and ga,* and *imitates sounds* such as a *cough, tongue-click, or razz.*

He is *persistent for toys* that are *out of his reach.* He gets his *feet to his mouth* while supine.

H	O	KEY AGE: 28 Weeks
		ADAPTIVE
		Cube, Bell: 1-hand approach & grasp
		2nd Cube: grasps 1st, grasps 2nd
		2nd Cube: grasps 2 more than momentarily
		3rd Cube: retains 2 as 3rd presented
		Massed Cubes: grasps 2 more than momentarily
		Cup & Massed Cubes: retains cube, grasps cup
		Cube, Bell, Ring-String: transfers adeptly
		Cube, Bell, Ring-String: bangs
		Bell: retains
		Ring-String: secures ring by string (*40w)
		GROSS MOTOR
		Sit: sits erect about 1 minute
		Stand: stands hands held (*32w)
		Prone: pivots (*36w)
		Prone: assumes creeping position
		Prone: crawls or creep-crawls (*36w)
		FINE MOTOR
		Cube: radial palmar grasp (*36w)
		Pellet: radial raking or unsuccessful inferior scissors grasp (*32w)
		String: inferior scissors grasp (*40w)
		LANGUAGE
		Vocalization: ah-ah-ah, oh-oh-oh, *not aaah* (*32w)
		Vocalization: mum-mum-mum, crying (*36w)
		Vocalization: single consonant sounds—da, ba, ga
		Vocalization: imitates sounds—cough, tongue-click, razz
		PERSONAL-SOCIAL
		Play: feet to mouth, supine
		Play: persistent for toys out of reach
		Play: bites & chews

EXAMINATION SEQUENCE

Sitting (Chair)

Situation No. *

24–28–32 Weeks

	Situation No.
Chair—Tabletop	7,8,9
Cubes 1,2,3	11
Massed Cubes	17
Cup and Cubes	20
Pellet	22
Pellet in Bottle	26
Yarn	5
Bird Call, Bell-Ring	24
Bell	25
Ring-String	32
Mirror	62
Sitting Supported	63
Standing Supported	65
Prone	1
(Supine)	3
(Rattle)	4
(Social Stimulation)	6
(Pull-to-Sitting)	

Italicized items appear for the first time in this sequence.

*Situation number identifies the examination situation described in Chapter 4, Examination Procedures.

( ) = Situation sometimes omitted for special reasons.

H = History
O = Observation
(*) = Pattern replaced by more mature one at later age.

2nd Cube: grasps 2 prolongedly
Massed Cubes: grasps 2 prolongedly
Cubes: hits, pushes cube with cube (*56w)
Cup & Massed Cubes: removes cube from cup
Pellet & Bottle: regards pellet if drops or thrown out

GROSS MOTOR

Sit: sits steady 10 minutes
Sit: leans forward, reerects (*36w)
Stand: holds rail, full weight (*48w)

FINE MOTOR

Pellet: inferior scissors grasp (*36w)

LANGUAGE

Vocalization: da-da or equivalent as sound (*36w)
Comprehension: responds to "no-no," tone of voice (*40w)
Comprehension: understands name; word, not voice
Communication: uses gesture

PERSONAL-SOCIAL

Feeding: feeds self cracker
Feeding: some milk from cup or glass
Social: plays peek-a-boo

ADAPTIVE

Rattle: 2-hand approach & grasp (*28w)
Rattle: shakes actively
Rattle: reaches after dropped rattle
Cube: 2-hand approach & grasp (*28w)
Cube, Bell: to mouth
Cubes: resecures dropped cube
Massed Cubes: grasps 1st, grasps 2nd
Massed Cubes: exploits 3 cubes
Cup & Massed Cubes: retains cube, regards cup (*28w)
Yarn: looks for fallen yarn

GROSS MOTOR

Supine: lifts head from platform
Supine: rolls to prone
Pull-to-sit: lifts head, assists (*36w)
Chair: trunk erect (*36w)
Sit: well, leaning on hands (*28w)
Stand: bounces (*28w)

FINE MOTOR

Cube: palmar grasp (*28w)
Pellet: contacts, rakes with whole hand (*28w)
String: contacts, rakes with whole hand (*28w)

LANGUAGE

Bird Call, Bell-Ring: turns head
Expressive: displeasure by sound other than crying (*——)

PERSONAL-SOCIAL

Feeding: takes solids well
Social: creates social contact
Social: pushes mother's hand away (*——)
Play: grasps feet, supine
Play: sits propped 30 minutes (*36w)
Mirror: pats mirror image

24 Weeks

ADAPTIVE

Rattle: 2-hand approach and grasp. Uses both hands in direct response to sight of rattle in supine. (See 28 weeks.)

Rattle: shakes actively. Distinguish active shaking by infant from passive sound of rattle as arms move.

Rattle: reaches after dropped rattle. When rattle falls or is removed and placed in sight on crib, infant reaches toward it and may roll to resecure it.

Cube: 2-hand approach and grasp. Uses both hands in direct response to sight of small object in sitting. (See 28 weeks.)

Cube, Bell: to mouth. Infant secures object by self and takes object, not back of hand, to mouth.

Cubes: resecures dropped cube. From massed or single cube situations; analogous to resecuring dropped rattle.

Massed Cubes: grasps 1st, grasps 2nd. Infant secures 1st cube by self and definitely reaches for and secures a 2nd at some point during manipulation.

Massed Cubes: exploits 3 cubes. During entire situation infant manages to grasp 3 different cubes.

Cup and Massed Cubes: retains cube, regards cup. Infant secures cube by self and retains that cube while looking at cup brought in from far edge of tabletop.

Yarn: looks for fallen yarn. As yarn moves across tabletop and drops off edge, infant not only turns head after fallen yarn but definitely looks down to where yarn has disappeared.

GROSS MOTOR

Supine: lifts head from platform. As though straining to sit up without assistance; from a completely flat position, not from semireclining position in infant carrier. Usually obtained by history.

Supine: rolls to prone. Gets both arms out from under chest after rolling completely over from back to abdomen.

Pull-to-Sitting: lifts head, assists. Flexes elbows and lifts head as soon as examiner's pull begins.

Chair: trunk erect. When securely strapped in, infant does not slump to side; reerects if leans toward tabletop in reaching.

Sitting: sits well, leaning on hands. Trunk straight, *maintaining* angle of at least 45° with crib, arms extended as props to prevent sagging forward. Surface should be *hard*. (See 28 weeks.)

Standing: bounces. When knees flex, infant extends them again. Examiner continues to provide support by keeping hands on chest below armpits.

FINE MOTOR

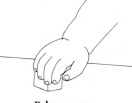

Palmar grasp

Cube: palmar grasp. Secures cube by self and holds it in center of palm, fingers closed around it. Whole hand grasp without radial differentiation. (See 28 weeks.)

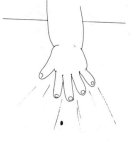

Rakes with whole hand

Pellet: contacts, rakes with whole hand. Hand over or near pellet, all fingers flexing in a raking, scratching movement; whole arm moves. Infant may succeed in touching pellet.

String: contacts, rakes with whole hand. (See above definition.)

LANGUAGE

Bird Call, Bell-Ring: turns head. In response to auditory cue, looks for source instead of merely altering activity.

Expressive: displeasure by sound other than crying. Expresses anger or unhappiness by sound that definitely is not crying.

PERSONAL-SOCIAL

Feeding: takes solids well. No longer extrudes baby food with tongue; food no longer needs wiping off chin.

Social: creates social contact. Initiates social contact by reaching out for or pulling at person.

Social: pushes mother's hand away. Uses hands or arms to push mother's hand away when she washes faces, wipes nose, etc., rather than just turning head or squirming.

Play: grasps feet, supine. Must be able to lift legs in extension to do this; grasps feet, not thighs.

Play: sits propped 30 minutes. May succeed tied in high chair or in corner of sofa or crib; needs less assistance from pillows than previously.

Mirror: pats mirror image. Definite regard for own face or hand, not merely random fingering of mirror itself.

28 Weeks

ADAPTIVE

Cube, Bell: 1-hand approach and grasp. Infant freed from symmetric postures. Approach and grasp synthesized in single coordinated movement in direct response to visual stimulus. (See 24 weeks.)

Second Cube: grasps 1st, grasps 2nd. After securing 1st by self, picks up 2nd cube presented.

Second Cube: grasps 2 more than momentarily. Holds 2 cubes secured by self for more than few seconds.

Third Cube: retains 2 as 3rd presented. Holds 2 cubes secured by self and retains them when 3rd is brought in from far edge of tabletop.

Massed Cubes: grasps 2 more than momentarily. Same definition as 2nd cube, above.

Cup and Massed Cubes: retains cube, grasps cup. Retains cube grasped by self and grasps cup when it is brought in from far edge of tabletop.

Cube, Bell, Ring-String: transfers adeptly. Smooth coordinated movements directly from one hand to other without intermediary of mouth or tabletop. Grasping hand does not pull object out of releasing hand, fingers do not get caught in each other.

Cube, Bell, Ring-String: bangs. Definite up-and-down vertical movement on tabletop.

Bell: retains. Maintains grasp; must engage in active banging or transfer.

Ring-String: secures ring by string. Hand contacts string on presentation or after reaching for ring first; in course of manipulation of string, ring comes within reach. Connection between ring and string not recognized. (See 40 weeks.)

GROSS MOTOR

Sitting: sits erect about 1 minute. On a *hard* surface, sits with back straight and maintains both hands up. (See 24 weeks.)

Standing: stands hands held. Infant's arms fully extended at shoulder height for balance only, not support, as hands are held. Body fully erect.

Prone: pivots. Moves in a circular manner on abdomen, by coordinated action of arms, usually crossing one over other.

Prone: assumes creeping position. Manages to get on hands and knees.

Prone: crawls or creep-crawls. Crawls forward while flat on abdomen ("army crawl"). *Creep-crawls:* gets on hands and knees, falls forward to abdomen and repeats these movements. (See 36 weeks.)

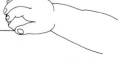

Radial palmar grasp

Cube: radial palmar grasp. Cube secured in palm of hand but off center, toward radial side; fingers closed about cube, thumb opposing them. (See 24 and 36 weeks.)

Pellet: radial raking or unsuccessful inferior scissors grasp. Radial raking—radial side of hand definitely oriented to pellet and takes lead in raking at pellet; less arm movement than at 24 weeks. Unsuccessful inferior scissors—infant attempts to grasp pellet by approximating thumb to *side* of index finger; other fingers curled and actively flexing simultaneously.

String: inferior scissors grasp. Infant succeeds in grasping string, as described above. String easier to secure in this fashion than pellet. (See 40 weeks.)

LANGUAGE

Vocalization: ah-ah-ah, oh-oh-oh, not *aah.* An advance over cooing which repeats same drawn-out vowel sound. Vocalizes same distinct syllables with control, or diverse vowel sounds in varying combinations, *e.g.,* ah-ah-ah, ah-oh-oh-oh, oh-uh-oh.

Vocalization: mum-mum-mum, crying. First active modulation of airstream with lips, usually while crying. Not a humming mmmm . . . ; a break in "M" sound is necessary.

Vocalization: single consonant sounds—da, ba, ga. Definite consonant syllable. May be preceded by vowel, *e.g.,* ah-da, but with stress on consonant.

Vocalization: imitates sounds—cough, tongue-click, razz: Repeats sounds, not words, initiated by mother.

PERSONAL-SOCIAL

Play: feet to mouth, supine. Gets feet into mouth.

Play: persistent for toys out of reach. May be at tabletop, in prone or in supine positions (usually rolls to prone).

Play: bites and chews. Definite up-and-down chomping movements. Distinguish from mouthing and licking. (See 20 weeks.)

32 Weeks

ADAPTIVE

Second Cube: grasps 2 prolongedly. Secures both cubes by self and holds for more than a minute.

Massed Cubes: grasps 2 prolongedly. Same as 2nd cube, above.

Cubes: hits, pushes cube with cube. Pushes cube on table with one in hand. Distinguish definite intent from accidental contact as infant bangs cubes.

Cup and Massed Cubes: removes cube from cup. After seeing examiner drop one in, or one falls in accidentally.

Pellet and Bottle: regards pellet if drops or is thrown out. Definitely looks for pellet in response to sound of its falling or if trajectory catches eye.

GROSS MOTOR

Sitting: sits steady 10 minutes. Both hands used in play. Still apt to throw self backward unexpectedly and mother unwilling to leave infant unattended.

Sitting: leans forward, reerects. After reaching for object at least an
arms's length away, reerects completely and smoothly, without
pushing up step-wise with arms.

Standing: holds rail, full weight. When placed standing at rail maintains position without leaning chest against rail. Knows enough to
hold on.

FINE MOTOR

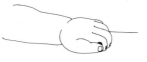

Inferior scissors grasp

Pellet: inferior scissors grasp. Succeeds in grasping pellet. (See 28
weeks.)

LANGUAGE

Vocalization: da-da or equivalent as sound. Definite combination of 2
or more consonant sounds, but without specific meaning. Ma-ma,
which usually comes later, qualifies. (See 36 and 40 weeks.)

Comprehension: responds to no-no, tone of voice. Pauses and looks at
person, but may subsequently continue activity. (See 40 weeks.)

Comprehension: understands name; word, not voice. Distinguishes
own name, rather than mere sound of person's voice. Does not respond in same way when someone else's name is called.

Communication: uses gesture. Initiates communication by reaching
out arms to be picked up by someone, shakes head for "no," etc.

PERSONAL-SOCIAL

Feeding: feeds self cracker. Eats whole cracker by successive purpose-
ful bites and munching, rather than simply sucking on it.

Feeding: some milk from cup or glass. Usually willing to accept water
and juice from cup at earlier age than willing to accept milk.
Mother holds cup.

Social: plays peek-a-boo. Engages in game by actively looking for person who hides, or initiates game by hiding own head. If plays by
pulling clothes off face, must be accompanied by a social response.

40 WEEKS

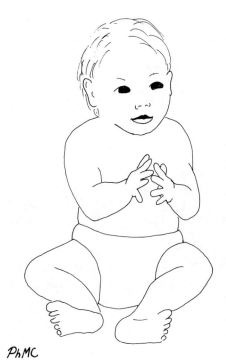

PhMC

Plays pat-a-cake

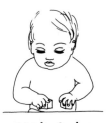

Matches 2 cubes

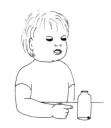

Points at pellet through glass

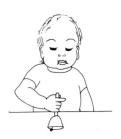

Grasps by handle

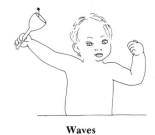

Waves

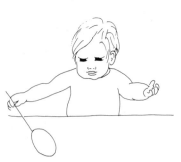

Sees connection, pulls string

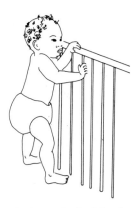

Cruises, using both hands

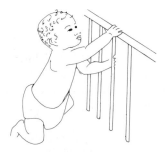

Lets self down with control

The 40-week-old infant sits before the table with good postural control, without support. After the introductory toy is removed, she gives immediate regard to the FIRST CUBE and seizes it with a radial digital grasp. She grasps the SECOND CUBE in a similar manner, holds them and brings the *two cubes into opposition,* looking at them as she *matches* them in her hands.

In the massed CUBES situation she approaches the mass immediately and again brings two cubes into combination. She exploits the cubes with method and control and may put them down with crude release, taking her hand off.

When the examiner places the CUP alongside the cluster of CUBES, she brings the cube she is holding against the outside of the cup. The examiner gestures, requesting the infant to put the cube into the cup, and drops one in if there is no response. The infant takes the cube out and then may thrust hand and cube into the cup but not let go.

For the CUBE AND PAPER situation, the examiner removes all but one cube and, while the infant watches, covers it with a piece of onionskin paper. She occasionally uncovers the toy to find it.

She approaches the PELLET with the extended index finger. Her arm rests on the table, and she *prehends the pellet promptly with an inferior pincer grasp.* The examiner then presents the PELLET BESIDE THE BOTTLE and calls attention to the pellet before bringing both in simultaneously. The infant may approach the pellet first but grasps the bottle, then picks up the pellet while holding the bottle. Holding the bottom of the bottle at the infant's eye level the examiner drops the pellet into the bottle and places the bottle on the table. The baby definitely sees THE PELLET IN THE BOTTLE and *points at it with her finger*.

The PEGBOARD is presented and the examiner inserts each peg in turn. Eventually the infant may remove some of the pegs from the pegboard by pulling them sideways before lifting them out.

She approaches the BELL and *grasps it by the handle*. She *waves* the bell, spontaneously or after demonstration, then *pokes at the clapper* as if to discover what makes the noise, in further demonstration of her interest in detail.

The RING-STRING, with the string within easy reach, is placed on the table. She looks back and forth from ring to string and *sees the connection* between them. In her eagerness to get the ring, she secures the string with a *scissors grasp*.

When the FORMBOARD is placed in front of the infant and she is handed the round block, she may bang or release it near the round hole after the examiner requests and demonstrates. Occasionally she removes it easily after the examiner has placed it.

The table is removed and the infant is placed close to the large MIRROR. She socializes with herself and looks back and forth from her image to the examiner's. The infant has already displayed her ability to SIT with good control. Enticed by a lure, she goes directly from sitting to prone, CREEPS forward on hands and knees with alternating movements, then pulls herself to standing at the railing. Holding the RAILING, she *cruises along using two hands*. She *retrieves a toy from the platform* with one hand while maintaining her support on the rail with the other and *lets herself down* from the rail with *good control*. She may WALK SUPPORTED with both hands held to provide balance only.

Her reported language behavior indicates that she vocalizes *da-da with meaning* and has a total of *two "words."* She *responds to the word "no-no,"* not just to the tone of voice. She plays *one nursery trick* such as bye-bye, pat-a-cake or peek-a-boo, *on verbal request* alone, showing she knows what the words mean.

In SOCIAL play she is reported to *imitate three nursery games* in response to her mother's demonstration, and *push her arms through a sleeve* once started to help in dressing. She *extends a toy* and may release it in response to request and gesture.

During the examination she no longer is confined to the tabletop and runs toys *along the crib rail*, drops them over the edge, or takes them down to the *crib platform* to play with them.

EXAMINATION SEQUENCE

Sitting (Crib)

	Situation No.*
36–40–44 Weeks	
Tabletop	
Cubes 1, 2, 3	7,8,9
Cubes	11
Cup and Cubes	17
Cube and Paper	18
Pellet	20
Pellet beside Bottle	21
Pellet in Bottle	22
Pegboard	27
Bell	24
Ring-String	25
Formboard	42
Mirror	32
Sitting Free	66
Prone	65
Railing	67
Walking Supported	68

Italicized items appear for the first time in this sequence.

*Situation number identifies the examination situation described in Chapter 4, Examination Procedures.

H = History
O = Observation
(*) = Pattern replaced by more mature one at later age.

H	O	KEY AGE: 40 Weeks
		ADAPTIVE
		Cubes: matches 2 cubes (*56w)
		Pellet & Bottle: points at pellet through glass (*15m)
		Bell: grasps by handle
		Bell: waves
		Bell: pokes at clapper
		Ring-String: sees connection, pulls string
		GROSS MOTOR
		Rail: cruises, using 2 hands (*44w)
		Rail: retrieves toy from floor (*52w)
		Rail: lets self down with control
		FINE MOTOR
		Pellet: grasps promptly
		Pellet: inferior pincer grasp (*48w)
		String: scissors grasp (*48w)
		LANGUAGE
		Vocabulary: da-da with meaning
		Vocabulary: any 2 "words"
		Comprehension: performs 1 nursery trick on verbal request
		Comprehension: responds to "no-no," word
		PERSONAL-SOCIAL
		Social: imitates 3 nursery tricks
		Social: extends toy, no release (*44w)
		Play: toys to side rail or platform (*52w)
		Dress: pushes arms through if started (*30m)

H	O	36 Weeks	H	O	44 Weeks

44 Weeks

ADAPTIVE
- Cup & Cubes: cube into cup, no release (*48w)
- Cube & Paper: uncovers cube (toy)
- Pellet & Bottle: approaches pellet first
- Formboard: removes round block easily
- Formboard: bangs or releases round block near hole (*48w)

GROSS MOTOR
- Sit: pivots in sitting
- Walks: 2 hands held (*48w)
- Rail: cruises, using 1 hand (*52w)

FINE MOTOR
- Cube: crude release (*56w)
- String: plucks promptly
- Pegboard: removes large round eventually (*52w)
- Pegboard: removes small round eventually (*52w)
- Pegboard: removes large square eventually (*52w)

LANGUAGE
- Vocabulary: ma-ma with meaning
- Vocabulary: any 3 "words"
- Vocalization: incipient jargon
- Comprehension: performs 2 nursery tricks on verbal request
- Comprehension: follows simple commands on verbal request

PERSONAL-SOCIAL
- Social: gives a toy, request and gesture
- Dress: lifts feet in dressing (*30m)

36 Weeks

ADAPTIVE
- Cup & Cubes: hits cube against cup (*44w)
- Pellet: index finger approach
- Pellet & Bottle: holds bottle, grasps pellet (*52w)

GROSS MOTOR
- Sit: indefinitely steady
- Sit: to prone with ease
- Prone: creeps on hands & knees (*56w)
- Prone: to sitting
- Stand: pulls to feet at rail (*52w)
- Rail: lifts, replaces foot (*52w)

FINE MOTOR
- Cube: radial digital grasp
- Pellet: scissors grasp (*40w)

LANGUAGE
- Vocabulary: any 1 "word"
- Vocalization: ma-ma as sound (*44w)
- Vocalization: "sings" along with music

PERSONAL-SOCIAL
- Feeding: holds own bottle (*21m)
- Social: imitates 2 nursery tricks

36 Weeks

ADAPTIVE

Cup and Cubes: hits cube against cup. Hits or brings cube in hand against cup; may even contact inside of cup. Distinguish intent from accidental contact.

Pellet: index finger approach. Essential feature is differentiation of or poking with index finger. May be exhibited with objects other than pellet.

Pellet and Bottle: holds bottle, grasps pellet. Picks up pellet while holding bottle. Is aware of smaller object and of 2 objects simultaneously.

GROSS MOTOR

Sitting: indefinitely steady. Uses both hands in play. Will not fall over if left alone in room. This is *the definition of sitting alone.*

Sitting: to prone position with ease. Goes directly and smoothly forward over feet from sitting, with good control.

Prone: creeps on hands and knees. On hands and knees, or hands and feet, trunk raised. Pulling self about on buttocks in sitting position (hitching) is locomotor variant roughly equivalent to creeping in maturity value. The meanings of creeping and crawling vary with geographic locale, so precise definition is necessary. (See 28 weeks.)

Prone: to sitting position. Goes from abdomen to sitting position with control.

Standing: pulls to feet at rail. Attains fully erect position.

Railing: lifts, replaces foot. In preparation for cruising, but without sidewise progression; 1 foot or each alternately.

FINE MOTOR

Radial digital grasp

Cube: radial digital grasp. Cube held with ends of thumb, index and 3rd fingers. Space visible between cube and palm. (See 28 weeks.)

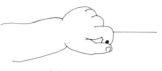

Scissors grasp

Pellet: scissors grasp. Successful prehension of pellet. (See 40 weeks, **String**.)

LANGUAGE

Vocabulary: any 1 "word." (See 40 weeks for definition of "word.")

Vocalization: ma-ma as sound. Combination of the 2 consonant sounds without specific meaning. (See 32 weeks.)

Vocalization: "sings" along with music. Definite vocalizing in response to music.

PERSONAL-SOCIAL

Feeding: holds own bottle. Retrieves dropped 8-ounce bottle and completes feeding with no assistance from mother.

Social: imitates 2 nursery tricks. Usually 1 nursery trick in addition to peek-a-boo, such as bye-bye or pat-a-cake. (See 32 and 40 weeks.)

40 Weeks

ADAPTIVE

Cubes: matches 2 cubes. Brings them together as though comparing them, or in pat-a-cake fashion. Both cubes grasped and usually lifted, and infant watches what is happening. Differentiate from pushing 1 cube with another. (See 32 weeks.)

Pellet and Bottle: points at pellet through glass. Looks at pellet while poking at it in the bottle.

Bell: grasps by handle. Indicates awareness of 2 distinct parts. Hand does not touch bowl at all. Initial grasp only.

Bell: waves. Distinguish active movement to produce sound from passive ringing as arms move; also differentiate from banging. Must be in sitting position, as distinct from shaking rattle while supine. (See 28 weeks.)

Bell: pokes at clapper. Visual fixation accompanies exploration. Distinguish from accidental contact of clapper during course of manipulation.

Ring-String: sees connection, pulls string. On first approach, indicates awareness that ring will be obtained by pulling on string; watches ring come in as pulls. (See 28 weeks.)

GROSS MOTOR

Railing: cruises, using 2 hands. Sideward walking, holding rail for support, shifting hands.

Railing: retrieves toy from floor. While standing and holding railing or furniture, bends down, retrieves toy and reerects to full standing position.

Railing: lets self down with control. Definitely takes care to let self down slowly rather than letting go and dropping abruptly.

FINE MOTOR

Pellet: grasps promptly. Independent of type of grasp, but secures consistently on 1st or 2nd approach. Usually not prompt if thumb and fingers not coordinated precisely.

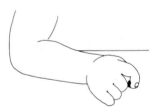

Inferior pincer grasp

Pellet: inferior pincer grasp. Between ventral surfaces of thumb and index (or middle) finger. Hand and arm resting on table surface provide accessory support. (See 48 weeks.)

String: scissors grasp. Successful prehension between thumb and *side* of index finger. Remaining ulnar fingers completely suppressed; are held loosely curled but do not flex and extend during prehension. The action of the last 3 fingers is what differentiates an "inferior scissors" from a "scissors" grasp. (See 28 weeks and narrative.)

LANGUAGE

Vocabulary: da-da with meaning. This or equivalent sound used specifically to refer to father. (See 32 weeks.)

Vocabulary: any 2 "words." "Word" is sound used consistently to refer to a person, action, object or group of objects, even if not recognizably articulated.

Comprehension: performs 1 nursery trick on verbal request. Understands what mother says when she uses words, and responds appropriately. May flex fingers for bye-bye, pat mother's arm for pat-a-cake, etc. (See Personal-Social below.)

Comprehension: responds to no-no, word. Infant responds just to word itself when harsh sound is not used. Distinguish between tone of voice and actual word. (See 32 weeks.)

PERSONAL-SOCIAL

Social: imitates 3 nursery tricks. Engages in nursery games if mother demonstrates first. Social play is distinct from comprehension. It also must be distinguished from self-initiated stereotyped patterning unrelated to social demand. (See Language above.)

Social: extends toy, no release. Spontaneously, or in response to extended hand and "Give it to me," "Thank-you," etc.

Play: toys to side rail or platform. No longer restricted to exploitation on tabletop only. Bangs toys on side rail of crib or runs them along it. Brings toys down from tabletop to platform with intent, and exploits objects on platform. Does not include simple restoring of dropped object from platform to table.

Dressing: pushes arms through if started. Aids in dressing and completes pushing arms through sleeves.

44 Weeks

ADAPTIVE

Cup and Cubes: cube into cup, no release. Thrusts hand holding cube inside cup but does not let go. Distinguish intent from accidental contact with inside of cup.

Cube and Paper: uncovers cube (toy). After examiner covers toy with paper while infant watches, infant definitely takes paper off to find toy. Distinguish intent from playing with paper after securing it or from accidental swiping of paper.

Pellet and Bottle: approaches pellet first. Reaches toward pellet first when both objects are presented simultaneously, although bottle may be grasped first.

Formboard: removes round block easily. Essential feature is awareness of how block has to be manipulated to remove it. Usually accomplished by lifting one edge with thumb and getting underneath block; occasionally holds hand over entire block, if hand is large enough.

Formboard: bangs or releases round block near hole. Indicates awareness that round block belongs in hole by looking at hole selectively and bringing block near it, banging or even releasing it near round hole.

GROSS MOTOR

Sitting: pivots in sitting. Moves in circular manner, swinging around on buttocks and using feet only to propel self. Does not turn whole body to reach to side.

Walks: 2 hands held. Infant's hands held for *balance only;* moves legs coordinately with forward impetus; trunk does not need support. Distinguish between infant walking and mother executing forward motion and sustaining infant's weight.

Railing: cruises, using 1 hand. Sideward walking, lifting and replacing hand on rail to progress.

FINE MOTOR

Cube: crude release. Puts cube down on tabletop and takes hand off, or releases cube into cup. As opposed to dropping, is a somewhat clumsy and exaggerated letting go.

String: plucks promptly. Consistently secures on 1st or 2nd approach, using ventral surfaces of thumb and one finger. Prompt but cruder grasp is not plucking.

Pegboard: removes large round eventually. Manages to take peg out after many attempts. Pulls at peg sideways. (See 52 weeks.)

Pegboard: removes small round eventually. Same as above.

Pegboard: removes large square eventually. Same as above.

LANGUAGE

Vocabulary: ma-ma with meaning. This or equivalent sound is used specifically to refer to mother. (See 36 weeks.)

Vocabulary: any 3 "words." See 40 weeks for definition of "word."

Vocalization: incipient jargon. Jargon is distinguished from baby babbling by presence of inflections and pauses. It sounds like a foreign language. At this age the jargon consists only of 2 or 3 word-like phrases. (See 52 weeks.)

Comprehension: performs 2 nursery tricks on verbal request. (See 40 weeks.)

Comprehension: follows simple commands on verbal request. Responds appropriately to requests such as "Sit down," "Come here," etc., without gestures being used.

PERSONAL-SOCIAL

Social: gives a toy, request and gesture. Places and actively releases into a person's hand, rather than merely permitting its removal. May be unwilling to part with favorite objects.

Dressing: lifts feet in dressing. Assists by lifting feet for shoes or diaper.

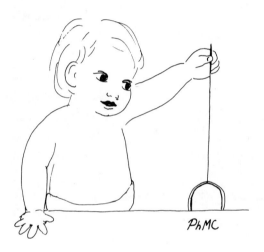

Dangles ring

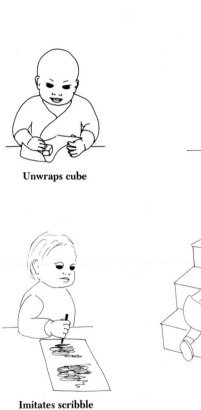

Unwraps cube

Inserts pellet

Imitates scribble

Creeps up

Pats pictures

Points for wants

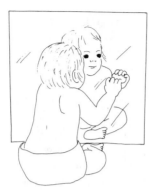

Offers toy to image

The 52-week-old child sits erect and unsupported before the table or on his mother's lap at an adjustable table. The introductory toy is removed tactfully as the PICTURE BOOK is placed on the table and the examiner starts to turn pages and comment on the pictures. The child *pats the pictures* and *helps to turn the pages.*

The FIRST, SECOND and THIRD CUBES are presented in succession. He may bring the cubes together briefly or try to pick them all up at once.

The examiner builds a TOWER OF TWO cubes and tries by demonstration and gesture to induce the child to do likewise. He tries to build on one of his own cubes or takes a cube from the model and attempts the tower. Most of the time, the tower falls when he releases the cube.

In the massed CUBES situation, he exploits cubes in a controlled manner. The CUP is placed alongside the cluster of CUBES. It is added soon after the mass of cubes, as this age tends to see the burgeoning of the new-found skill of casting. The examiner then requests and gestures to induce the child to put a cube into the cup. He *puts* as many as *five cubes into the cup,* although demonstration may be necessary. The examiner may offer cubes sequentially to the child's hand to encourage the task.

After the child succeeds in discovering the CUBE under the CUP, which he has watched the examiner hide, the examiner proceeds with the CUBE AND PAPER situation. After watching the examiner wrap the cube completely in a piece of onionskin paper, the child definitely *unwraps the paper to* secure the cube.

Presented with the PELLET BESIDE THE BOTTLE, he reaches for the pellet first and picks it up with a neat pincer grasp. The examiner points to the bottle and gently inhibits the child's taking the pellet to his mouth. After the examiner requests and gestures, or perhaps demonstrates, the child *inserts the* PELLET IN THE BOTTLE. He is interested in the *pellet only, unless it is inside the bottle.*

The PEGBOARD is presented and the pegs are inserted successively in their respective holes. The child *removes all pegs with ease by* lifting them out of the holes without pulling them sideways. He may insert the large round eventually.

In the RING-STRING situation, with the string within reach, he reaches immediately for the end of the string, plucks it easily and secures the ring. He *dangles the ring* by the string, or he may decide it is too simple for his level of sophistication and cast it away.

When the examiner DRAWS vigorously back and forth at the top of a piece of paper, and then hands the crayon to the child, he SCRIBBLES *imitatively.* He sometimes tries to make a stroke in imitation of the examiner's decisive VERTICAL STROKE.

He pulls at the FORMBOARD which is presented with the round hole at the right and the triangular hole in front of the child's chest. The examiner holds the board in place and offers the child the round block. Demonstration may be needed before the child inserts it in the correct hole. He occasionally adapts to rotation of the board if the examiner points to the correct hole.

The TOY AND STICK are presented, the toy placed out of the child's reach but within reach of the stick. The child sometimes tries to get the toy with the stick after the examiner has demonstrated.

The table then is removed and the BALL is offered. He accepts the ball and on invitation gives it to the examiner, who tosses the ball so that it bounces a bit towards the child. The child engages in cooperative ball play and *releases* the ball *with a good cast.*

Before the MIRROR he looks from his image to the examiner's image. He accepts and retains the ball placed in his hands, and *offers it to his mirror image.*

His WALKING includes *rising independently* in the middle of the floor, then *taking several steps.* While STANDING he bends to *pick up an object from the floor* without holding on. He is reported to *climb into a* SMALL CHAIR *and sit,* and occasionally succeed in climbing into an ADULT CHAIR. He *creeps up* STAIRS.

His language includes six *"words"* and *jargon.* He also is reported to look at named objects and may get a familiar toy from another room. He *points specifically for his wants, casts toys in play or refusal,* and *hugs a doll or stuffed animal.*

EXAMINATION SEQUENCE

Sitting (Crib)

H	O	KEY AGE: 52 Weeks	48–52–56 Weeks	Situation No.*
		ADAPTIVE	Tabletop	
		Cup & Cubes: releases 5 cubes in cup	*Picture Book*	46
		Cube & Paper: unwraps cube (toy)	Cubes 1, 2, 3	7,8,9
		Pellet & Bottle: takes pellet only, unless inside bottle	Tower 2	10
		Pellet & Bottle: inserts pellet	Cubes	11
		Draw: imitates scribble (*15m)	Cup and Cubes	17
		Ring-String: dangles ring by string	Cup and Cube	19
			Cube and Paper	18
		GROSS MOTOR	Pellet beside Bottle	21
		Stand: picks up object from floor	Pellet in Bottle	22
		Walks: rises independently, takes several steps (*15m)	Pegboard	27
		Stairs: creeps up (*15m)	Ring-String	25
		Small Chair: climbs into and sits	*Drawing: Scribble Imitation*	35
			Vertical Stroke	36
		FINE MOTOR	Formboard	42
		Picture Book: helps turn pages (*18m)	*Toy and Stick*	28
		Pegboard: removes all pegs with ease	*Small Ball: Ball Play*	58
		Ball: releases with good cast	*Mirror and Ball*	33
			Sitting Free	66
		LANGUAGE	Railing	67
		Vocabulary: 6 "words"	Walking Supported	68
		Vocalization: uses jargon	*Walking*	70
		Picture Book: pats picture (*15m)	*Stairs*	71
		PERSONAL-SOCIAL		
		Communication: points for wants (*——)		
		Play: casts in play or refusal		
		Play: hugs doll or stuffed animal		
		Mirror: offers toy to image		

Italicized items appear for the first time in this sequence

*Situation number identifies the examination situation described in Chapter 4, Examination Procedures.

H = History
O = Observation
(*) = Pattern replaced by more mature one at later age.

H	O	48 Weeks	H	O	56 Weeks
		ADAPTIVE			**ADAPTIVE**
		Cubes: tries tower, fails (*56w)			Cubes: tower of 2
		Cup & Cubes: releases 2 cubes in cup			Cup & Cubes: releases 9 in cup
		Cup & Cube: picks up cup to discover cube (toy)			Draw: incipient imitation stroke (*18m)
		Pellet & Bottle: grasps pellet first			Toy & Stick: tries to get toy with stick, demonstration (*15m)
		Pellet & Bottle: tries inserting, fails (*52w)			Formboard: inserts round block, no demonstration
		Formboard: inserts round block, demonstration (*56w)			Formboard: adapts to rotation with pointing (*15m)
		GROSS MOTOR			**GROSS MOTOR**
		Stand: momentarily alone, maintaining balance (*52w)			Walks: creeping discarded
		Walks: 1 hand held (*52w)			Walks: squats in play
		Walks: few steps from object to object (*52w)			Adult Chair: climbs into
		FINE MOTOR			**FINE MOTOR**
		Pellet: neat pincer grasp			Cubes: tower of 2
		Pegboard: removes small square eventually (*52w)			Pegboard: inserts large round eventually (*15m)
		Ball: releases with slight cast (*52w)			
		LANGUAGE			**LANGUAGE**
		Vocabulary: 4 "words"			Vocabulary: 8 "words"
		Comprehension: looks at named inanimate objects			Comprehension: gets object from another room
		PERSONAL–SOCIAL			**PERSONAL–SOCIAL**
		Ball: cooperative ball play			

GLOSSARY

48 Weeks

Cubes: tries tower, fails. Tower falls when cube is released on top of one on tabletop. Rarely, tower "built" in hands and tower cube held on.

Cup and Cubes: releases 2 cubes in cup. Distinguish intent from accidental falling of cube into cup. (See 52 weeks.)

Cup and Cube: picks up cup to discover cube (toy). After examiner covers cube with cup while infant watches, infant definitely takes cup off to find cube. Distinguish intent from playing with cup after securing it, or from accidental swiping of cup.

Pellet and Bottle: grasps pellet first. Definitely prefers pellet and picks up pellet first when both objects presented simultaneously.

Pellet and Bottle: tries inserting, fails. Pellet falls outside bottle. It is not necessarily released over neck of bottle but definitely brought into relation with bottle and released. (See 52 weeks.)

Formboard: inserts round block, demonstration. Indicates perception of relationship after examiner inserts block, and places block completely in hole.

Standing: momentarily alone, maintaining balance. When infant lets go, does not fall immediately.

Walks: 1 hand held. Coordinated *forward*, not circular, drive when hand held for *balance only*, not support.

Walks: few steps from object to object. Infant takes steps between objects or people. Has to pull up or be placed in standing to achieve this. (See 52 weeks.)

Neat pincer grasp

Pellet: neat pincer grasp. The adult grasp between ventral surfaces of thumb and index (or middle) finger, hand and arm elevated above table surface. Discarding accessory support of arm or hand resting on tabletop is what distinguishes neat from inferior pincer grasp. (See 40 weeks.)

Pegboard: removes small square eventually. Manages to take peg out after many attempts. Pulls at peg sideways. (See 52 weeks.)

Ball: releases with slight cast. Succeeds in giving ball slight drop forward after many tries. Movement not smooth or coordinated.

LANGUAGE

Vocabulary: 4 "words." (See 52 weeks for definition of "word.")

Comprehension: looks at named inanimate objects. Infant *looks* at or goes to named object. Includes only inanimate objects, not persons or pets; bottle also excluded.

PERSONAL-SOCIAL

Ball: cooperative ball play. Indicates awareness of social situation and participates in social play by rolling or casting ball to examiner.

52 Weeks

ADAPTIVE

Cup and Cubes: releases 5 cubes in cup. May start to take cubes out after a few are put in, but eventually has 5 inside cup. Cannot complete task with all 10 cubes.

Cube and Paper: unwraps cube (toy). Child definitely opens up paper and unwraps cube to find it.

Pellet and Bottle: takes pellet only, unless inside bottle. Gives virtually exclusive attention to pellet. May pick up bottle if pellet is inside.

Pellet and Bottle: inserts pellet. Releases pellet into bottle. (See 48 weeks.)

Drawing: imitates scribble. Reproduction of the back-and-forth motion demonstrated by examiner, even though no marks appear on paper or tabletop surface is utilized.

Ring-String: dangles ring by string. Essential feature is awareness of relationship between ring and string. Distinguish between passive dangling of ring as arm moves, and active exploitation as child watches ring move up and down.

GROSS MOTOR

Standing: picks up object from floor. While standing independently, child bends down to secure toy from floor and stands up again.

Walks: rises independently, takes several steps. Child has enough control to get up in middle of floor by self, stop and start again without support, and catch self, if falling occurs. This is *the definition of walking alone.* (See 48 weeks).

Stairs: creeps up. Ascends more than 1 or 2 steps.

Small Chair: climbs into and sits. Any successful method that involves climbing in, turning around, and sitting down.

FINE MOTOR

Picture Book: helps turn pages. Child completes turning page the examiner has lifted halfway by pushing it down in proper direction. Uses book as book not merely another toy to manipulate.

Pegboard: removes all pegs with ease. Indicates awareness that pegs must be pulled straight up. Removes on 1st or 2nd attempt without sideways pulling. (See 48 weeks.)

Ball: releases with good cast. Smooth release is shown, although direction may not be accurate. Definite throwing motion.

LANGUAGE

Vocabulary: 6 "words." "Word" is sound used consistently to refer to a person, action, object or group of objects, even if not recognizably articulated.

Vocalization: uses jargon. Jargon is distinguished from baby babbling by presence of inflections and pauses. It sounds like sentences uttered in a foreign language. Is rich and elaborate, encompassing whole "sentences" and "paragraphs" by this age. (See 44 weeks.)

Picture Book: pats pictures. Distinguish from indiscriminate patting of tabletop.

PERSONAL-SOCIAL

Communication: points for wants. Indicates specific object desired. Usually accompanied by vocalization, but is not merely fussing until mother gets desired one from among many.

Play: casts in play or refusal. Definite throwing motion. A very characteristic pattern at this age which may interfere with other examination responses.

Play: hugs doll or stuffed animal. Hugs or loves stuffed toy.

Mirror: offers toy to image. Essential feature is offering ball to self, rather than merely bringing it against mirror.

56 Weeks

ADAPTIVE

Cubes: tower of 2. Releases 1 cube on top of another, and tower stands. (See 48 weeks.)

Cup and Cubes: releases 9 in cup. Eventually has 9 of 10 inside cup. Cannot complete job. (See 52 weeks.)

Drawing: incipient imitation stroke. In attempting to imitate stroke, child makes definite movement in air, which then may be followed by scribbling. Movement may be only in the air.

Toy and Stick: tries to get toy with stick, demonstration. After examiner demonstrates use of stick in getting toy, child definitely tries to get it but does not succeed.

Formboard: inserts round block, no demonstration. Inserts completely. into hole, spontaneously or after request or pointing.

Formboard: adapts to rotation with pointing. Child places round block correctly after formboard is rotated, if examiner points to correct hole. Child's attention may or may not be sustained enough to watch and complete several rotations.

GROSS MOTOR

Walks: creeping discarded. This implies walking is child's preferred method of locomotion; if speed or efficiency is desired there will not be reversion to the more primitive method. Under stress of fatigue, however, child may still creep occasionally.

Walks: squats in play. Rests on heels with sufficient control and balance so that position is maintained for several minutes while playing on floor or ground.

Adult Chair: climbs into. Child faces chair, climbs up, then turns around to sit down. Success influenced by relative sizes of child and chair.

FINE MOTOR

Cubes: tower of 2. Tower stands without assistance from examiner.

Pegboard: inserts large round eventually. After several attempts and awkward manipulation, manages to insert the large round peg. (See 18 months.)

LANGUAGE

Vocabulary: 8 "words." (See 52 weeks for definition of "word.")

Comprehension: gets object from another room. Understands mother's request and complies when asked to go into another room to get some familiar object—shoe, diaper, bottle, etc.

PERSONAL-SOCIAL

Not applicable.

18 MONTHS

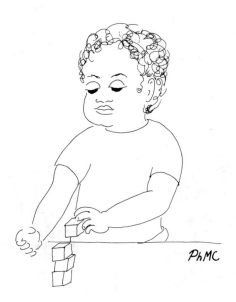

Tower of 4

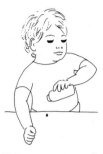

Dumps spontaneously

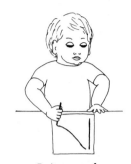

Imitates stroke

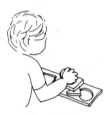

Piles 3 blocks

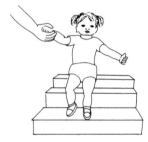

Walks down, 1 hand held

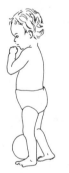

Walks into, steps on

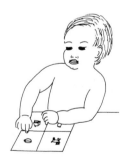

Points to 1

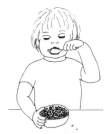

Inhibits turning spoon

The 18-month-old child has been WALKING well alone and RUN-NING stiffly without falling for a few months. She seats herself in the small chair before the table on which there is a bag of blocks, and the mother sits nearby to assist actively in her initial adjustment.

The PICTURE BOOK is placed on the table and the examiner starts to turn the pages and comment on the pictures. The child looks selectively at the pictures, *pointing to one* when requested, and *turns the pages two or three at a time.*

The CUBES then are presented, and when the child has begun to manipulate them, a TOWER of two to three cubes is demonstrated and requested. The child builds a *tower of four* cubes responsively. After the examiner has demonstrated a four-cube TRAIN, she responds *imitatively by pushing one or two cubes* along the table. She fills the CUP WITH CUBES without much urging, but when the examiner extends her hands and asks for the cup, she takes them out one by one or dumps them.

The PELLET AND BOTTLE are presented and the child inserts the pellet, spontaneously or on request. When asked to get it out, she *dumps the pellet* out of the bottle or *hooks it out* with her finger.

The PEGBOARD then is presented. After the examiner demonstrates, the child *inserts* the large and *small round* pegs *immediately* and *eventually* manages to *insert* the large and *small square* pegs.

The examiner shows the child a doll and asks her to identify eyes, nose, mouth, etc. The child *points to four* BODY PARTS either on herself, her mother, the examiner, or the doll.

For the DRAWING situation a blank piece of paper is placed on the table, a crayon is handed to the child and she scribbles *spontaneously*. After a decisive VERTICAL STROKE is demonstrated, she makes an *imitative stroke* without directional orientation.

The FORMBOARD is presented with the three blocks on the table, each one in front of its appropriate hole. The child either *puts a block near each hole*, although not necessarily the correct one, or *piles the three blocks* on the board or the table. After the examiner *demonstrates* correct placement, the child *inserts the three blocks*. She manages to *adapt to rotation* of the formboard, placing the blocks in the correct holes by trial and error *after the examiner points to each*.

The VERTICAL SLOT or PERFORMANCE BOX is presented and the child offered the square block. She brings it flat against the box or slot and, *after demonstration*, she finally is able to adjust the block and *insert it*.

The TOY AND STICK are presented with the toy out of the child's reach, but within reach of the stick. The child may try to get the toy without demonstration, but usually does not succeed until the examiner shows the technique.

The examiner presents the PICTURE CARD and asks the child to name the dog, shoe, cup, and house. If she does not respond, the examiner asks her to identify the pictures. The child names or *points correctly to one picture*. She may turn the card over or hand it back.

The child is shown four TEST OBJECTS (pencil, key, penny, and the examiner's shoe) in succession and asked to name them. Then the pencil, key, and penny are placed on the table in the child's reach and she is asked to give each in turn to the examiner. Following this, she is given the small ball. She *points correctly to two* of the objects, including *one* she has named, usually the ball.

The table then is moved slightly from its position and the child given free access to the room. On request she HURLS the SMALL BALL and *carries out two* of the following DIRECTIONS: "Put it on the table . . . On the chair . . . Give it to mother . . . To me." The child releases the ball IN the performance BOX or BASKET and reaches in, but is unable to solve the problem of turning it over and finally abandons the effort.

A LARGE BALL is placed on the floor and a kick is demonstrated. The child responds by *walking into or stepping on the ball* without giving it a true kick.

She *walks* up and *down* STAIRS *with one hand held,* and she has been *climbing on* a CHAIR *to reach things.*

Reported language behavior includes as many as *20–29 words, combining two different ideas in words,* and *calling playmates by name.* She is reported to *request food, drink* and *more,* and to *recognize a familiar TV theme, record or song.*

She *no longer turns the spoon over* before it gets to her mouth. She *hands the empty dish* when she is done and *handles a regular cup well,* putting it down when she is finished. She *imitates domestic chores,* such as dusting and hammering, and *puts a hat* on by herself. She is reported to *repeat the last two or more words* as she listens to someone else speaking.

EXAMINATION SEQUENCE

Locomoter (Child's Table and Chair)

15–18 Months	Situation No.*
Table and Chair	
Picture Book	46
Cubes: Tower	12
Train	13
Cup and Cubes	17
Pellet beside Bottle	21
Pegboard	27
Body Parts	47
Drawing: Spontaneous	34
Vertical Stroke	36
Formboard	42
Vertical Slot or Performance Box	43
Toy and Stick	28
Picture Card	48
Test Objects	52
Small Ball: Ball Play	58
Directions	59
In Basket or Performance Box	60
Large Ball	69
Walking, *Running*	70
Stairs	71

Italicized items appear for the first time in this sequence.
*Situation number identifies the examination situation described in Chapter 4, Examination Procedures.

H = **History**
O = **Observation**
(*) = **Pattern replaced by more mature one at later age.**

H	O	15 Months
		ADAPTIVE
		Cubes: tower of 3 Cup & Cubes: all into cup Pellet & Bottle: dumps, demonstration (*18m) Draw: spontaneous scribble Toy & Stick: gets toy with stick, demonstration (*24m) Formboard: adapts round block promptly after rotation Formboard: inserts square block, demonstration
		GROSS MOTOR
		Walks: alone, seldom falls Walks: fast, runs stiffly (*21m) Stairs: walks up, 1 hand held (*21m) Stairs: creeps down (*18m) Chair: climbs on to reach things Ball: hurls (*36m)
		FINE MOTOR
		Cubes: tower of 3 Pegboard: inserts large round immediately Pegboard: inserts small round eventually (*18m) Pegboard: inserts large square eventually (*24m)
		LANGUAGE
		Vocabulary: 10–19 words Picture Book: looks selectively (*18m) Body Parts: points to 1 Ball: follows 1 directional command
		PERSONAL-SOCIAL
		Feeding: leaves dish on tray Feeding: feeds self with spoon, spills (*18m) Communication: says "thank you" or equivalent Communication: seeks help in doing things Communication: pulls to show (*——) Play: pulls toy after self

H	O	KEY AGE: 18 Months
		ADAPTIVE
		Cubes: tower of 4 Cubes: imitates pushing train (*21m) Pellet & Bottle: dumps or hooks out spontaneously Draw: imitates stroke (*36m) Formboard: puts single blocks on or piles 3 (*24m) Formboard: inserts 3 blocks after demonstration (*24m) Formboard: adapts to rotation with pointing (*21m) Vertical Slot: inserts square block, demonstration (*21m)
		GROSS MOTOR
		Stairs: walks down, 1 hand held (*21m) Large Ball: walks into or steps on, demonstration (*21m)
		FINE MOTOR
		Cubes: tower of 4 Picture Book: turns 2–3 pages at once (*30m) Pegboard: inserts small round immediately Pegboard: inserts small square eventually (*24m)
		LANGUAGE
		Vocabulary: 20–29 words Speech: combines 2–3 words (*24m) Speech: calls playmates by name Communication: asks for more Communication: asks for food Communication: asks for drink Test Objects: names 1 Picture Book: points to 1 Picture Card: points to 1 Test Objects: points to 2 Body Parts: points to 4 Comprehension: recognizes TV theme, record, song Ball: follows 2 directional commands
		PERSONAL-SOCIAL
		Feeding: inhibits turning spoon (*24m) Feeding: hands empty dish Feeding: handles regular cup well Communication: echoes 2 or more last words (*——) Play: domestic mimicry Dress: puts on hat

15 Months

ADAPTIVE

Cubes: tower of 3. Successfully stacks 3 cubes; tower falls with 4th. (See 18 months.)

Cup and Cubes: all into cup. Puts all cubes in, spontaneously or with urging and demonstration. This implies that child completes the job.

Pellet and Bottle: dumps, demonstration. Intentionally turns bottle over after examiner demonstrates. (See 18 months.)

Drawing: spontaneous scribble. Makes definite marks on paper or tabletop, even if not vigorous or prolific. May do so only after asked to write on the paper by pointing and/or request.

Toy and Stick: gets toy with stick, demonstration. Child secures toy, pulling it close enough to pick up, after examiner shows use of stick.

Formboard: adapts round block promptly after rotation. Puts round block in correct hole promptly, either by correcting own error or by seeing correct placement immediately.

Formboard: inserts square block, demonstration. Puts square block in square hole after being shown by examiner. Examiner may assist in adjusting corners.

GROSS MOTOR

Walks: alone, seldom falls. Child walks well; losing balance is uncommon.

Walks: fast, runs stiffly. Unable to flex knees and coordinate arms in more mature pattern. Has difficulty stopping without barrier. (See 21 months.)

Stairs: walks up, 1 hand held. In erect position, not half-creeping. Adult provides balance only, not support.

Stairs: creeps down. More than 1 or 2 steps.

Chair: climbs on to reach things. Uses chair or stool to secure objects.

Ball: hurls. Throws in standing position without losing balance, with good cast. Younger child sits down to throw ball. Distinguish from dropping with slight cast.

FINE MOTOR

Cubes: tower of 3. Stands without assistance from examiner.

Pegboard: inserts large round immediately. (See 18 months for definition of "immediately.")

Pegboard: inserts small round eventually. (See 18 months for definition of "eventually.")

Pegboard: inserts large square eventually. (See 18 months.)

LANGUAGE

Vocabulary: 10–19 words. (See 18 months for definition of words.)

Picture Book: looks selectively. Follows examiner's hand as it moves from one detail to another and from one page to another. May put finger on details of picture, but not in response to examiner's request and without accompanying verbalization.

Body Parts: points to 1. Child puts finger on 1 body part. (See 18 months.)

Ball: follows 1 directional command. Complies on verbal request only. (See 18 months.)

PERSONAL–SOCIAL

Feeding: leaves dish on tray. Mother leaves dish on feeding surface, since child no longer is apt to throw it to floor.

Feeding: feeds self with spoon, spills. Eats part of meal with spoon, not fingers, without any direct help.

Communication: says "thank you" or equivalent. Any sounds that are used to mean it, on giving or receiving an object.

Communication: seeks help in doing things. Comes over to person and indicates help is needed in doing something, *e.g.*, showing toy to be wound up.

Communication: pulls to show. Takes mother's hand or dress and leads her to kitchen sink, as contrasted with standing at sink, pointing and vocalizing, etc. (See 52 weeks.)

Play: pulls toy after self. While creeping or walking; not sitting down and using string to secure attached toy, or using a handle to push a toy.

18 Months

ADAPTIVE

Cubes: tower of 4. Successfully stacks 4 cubes; tower falls with 5th. May need demonstration to begin and urging to continue. Examiner may assist with holding if child indicates intent to build by bringing successive cubes to tower, but has motor abnormality.

Cubes: imitates pushing train. Child pushes 1 or more cubes along tabletop after examiner demonstrates and then dismantles train. Distinguish imitation from rejection of situation by shoving cubes off table.

Pellet and Bottle: dumps or hooks out spontaneously. Intentionally turns bottle over. Distinguish from accidental dropping out as child shakes or manipulates bottle. Hooking pellet with finger (rare) is an equivalent response.

Drawing: imitates stroke. Makes definite stroke, without regard to direction. May be obliterated immediately by scribbling in an overproductive child. Stroke may be made on tabletop.

Formboard: puts single blocks on or piles 3. Places 1 block near each hole, not necessarily correct holes, or stacks 3 on formboard or table, as spontaneous response to initial presentation.

Formboard: inserts 3 blocks after demonstration. Places 3 blocks correctly at some time during the situation, after demonstration of the complete task. Examiner may help child adjust corners of square and triangle to fit.

Formboard: adapts to rotation with pointing. Places blocks correctly by trial and error after formboard is rotated, if examiner points to the proper holes.

Vertical Slot or Performance Box: inserts square block, demonstration. Adapts block completely to hole by trial and error.

GROSS MOTOR

Stairs: walks down, 1 hand held. In erect position. Adult provides balance only, not support.

Large Ball: walks into or steps on, demonstration. Contacts by stepping on or walking into, without foot swing. Holding on for support not permitted.

FINE MOTOR

Cubes: tower of 4. Tower stands without assistance from examiner.

Picture Book: turns 2 or 3 pages at once. Definite evidence of complete turn, in either direction, with inspection of pages; not random manipulation for its own sake.

Pegboard: inserts small round immediately. Indicates awareness of how the peg goes in and inserts small round smoothly on 1st or 2nd attempt.

Pegboard: inserts small square eventually. After several attempts and awkward manipulation, manages to insert small square peg.

Vocabulary: 20–29 words. Words have begun to acquire more specific meaning and include names of siblings, relatives, and friends. May be understood only by family members because of immature articulation.

Speech: combines 2 to 3 words. Implies 2 separate ideas. "Daddy go, bye mama, baby bed," are acceptable combinations. "All gone, what's that, big boy, oh dear," are essentially single words.

Speech: calls playmates by name. Does not have to be adult pronunciation.

Communication: asks for more. Usually accompanied by gesture in addition to word.

Communication: asks for food. By word—cookie, bread, fruit, etc.

Communication: asks for drink. By word—milk, water, juice, etc.

Test Objects: names 1. Pencil, key, penny, shoe, ball.

Picture Book: points to 1. Puts finger on or, if shy and wary, clearly looks at.

Picture Card: points to 1. Usually dog or shoe, as with picture book above.

Test Objects: points to 2. Total includes one already named correctly.

Body Parts: points to 4. Puts finger on part requested, on doll, own body, or mother's or examiner's body. Total includes those already named correctly, if any.

Comprehension: recognizes TV theme, record, song. Indicates recognition by running in to see TV when particular program is broadcast, heightens interest and attention when particular record is played, etc.

Ball: follows 2 directional commands. Complies on verbal request only. May throw ball at chair, table, mother or examiner, but not seat self on chair holding ball.

Feeding: inhibits turning spoon. Gets spoon to mouth right side up.

Feeding: hands empty dish. Gives dish for disposal when eating completed.

Feeding: handles regular cup well. Lifts, drinks, replaces. Younger child tilts cup too far, spilling profusely, or is apt to drop or throw cup when finished drinking.

Communication: echoes 2 or more last words. Repeats end of sentence adults have said.

Play: domestic mimicry. Imitates things mother or father does around house, *e.g.,* sweeping, dusting, hammering, etc.

Dressing: puts on hat. Succeeds in getting hat on head, not just setting it on top in any direction.

24 MONTHS

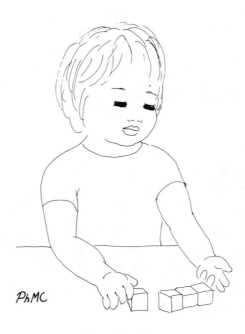

Aligns 4 for train

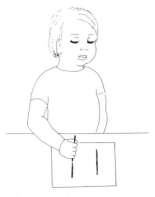

Imitates vertical stroke

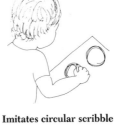

Imitates circular scribble

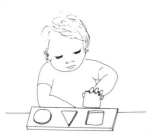

Inserts 3 blocks spontaneously

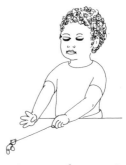

Attains toy, no demonstration

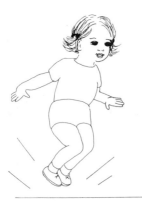

Jumps, both feet off floor

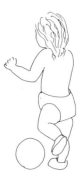

Kicks

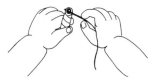

Threads shoelace through

The 2-year-old seats himself with ease and addresses himself at once to the PICTURE BOOK when it is placed on the table. He *names two pictures* and *identifies the correct action* on request.

The CUBES are presented, a "house" or TOWER requested, and demonstrated if necessary. Responsively, the child builds a *tower of seven cubes,* which falls with the eighth. He may be urged to make the tower "high." In imitation of a four-cube TRAIN, *he aligns all four,* and he may add the CHIMNEY to the train. He fills the CUP WITH CUBES and hands it to the examiner on request.

The PEGBOARD is presented, and the examiner places the large round peg. The child removes it easily and replaces it immediately. He then *inserts all* of the three remaining *pegs* in succession *promptly.*

The examiner demonstrates the insertion of the shoelace through the hole in the end of the SAFETY PIN. The child *threads the shoelace through,* although another demonstration from the examiner may be necessary.

The examiner shows the child a doll and asks him to name the eyes, nose, mouth, etc. He *names at least one* BODY PART and *points to the remaining six.*

When paper and crayon are presented for DRAWING the child scribbles SPONTANEOUSLY, but does not respond when asked what he has made. When a decisive VERTICAL STROKE is demonstrated, he *imitates the vertical stroke* with correct orientation. However, he is unable to alter his direction in imitation of a HORIZONTAL STROKE. A CIRCULAR SCRIBBLE then is demonstrated, and he *imitates the circular scribble,* differentiating it clearly from the vertical stroke and making several circles on top of each other.

The examiner now shows the PICTURE CARDS, and asks him to name the dog, shoe, house, clock, etc. After the child has named as many as he can, the examiner asks him to identify the rest. The child *names three,* and *points to seven pictures,* including those he already has named correctly.

The FORMBOARD is presented with each block in front of its appropriate hole. The child *inserts all of the blocks* in their correct holes *spontaneously.* The examiner now lifts the board and rotates it 180° to reverse the position of the holes. When asked to look at all the holes, the child learns to correct the initial errors he makes and adapts to the rotation.

The VERTICAL SLOT or PERFORMANCE BOX is presented and the child inserts the square block, adjusting the corners spontaneously.

The placard carrying the five red COLOR FORMS is placed on the table and the child is asked to place the circle, square, triangle, semicircle and cross, one after the other. If it is necessary to demonstrate the circle, he *places two* additional forms correctly.

The TOY AND STICK are presented, with the toy out of the child's reach but within reach of the stick. The child *gets the toy with the stick on request.*

He is shown the TEST OBJECTS (pencil, key, penny, examiner's shoe) in succession and asked to name them. He *names four* of them and may give the use of one or indicate the use of the key or penny. Following this he is given the ball.

The table is moved so that he may stand and walk about. He hurls the BALL on request and carries out all four of the following DIRECTIONS: "Put it on the table . . . On the chair . . . Give it to mother . . . To me." The ball is dropped into the PERFORMANCE BOX or BASKET and he gets it by tipping the box over or by crawling in to get it. If he is tall enough to reach the ball in the box, the situation is omitted.

A LARGE BALL is offered and the child asked to kick it. He *kicks* the ball on *verbal command alone,* swinging his foot against it.

His postural control is becoming facile, and he RUNS well, stopping himself at will. He JUMPS, getting *both feet off* the floor at the same time, and he is reported to *jump off the bottom step,* landing on both feet simultaneously. He tries to STAND *on one foot* without holding on. He walks up and down STAIRS alone, two feet to each step, holding the railing if necessary.

His mother estimates his vocabulary at well *over 50 words,* and *jargon* has been *replaced* by simple *three- or four-word sentences.* He uses the pronouns "*I*," "*you*," "*me*," and "*mine*." He soliloquizes, *verbalizing his immediate experiences, calling himself by pronouns* such as "I" and "me" ("Me slide . . . I fall down . . ."). He is reported to *use plurals* and *to fill in some words in familiar rhymes, songs, or TV commercials.*

His mother reports that he *feeds himself well with little spilling,* and *indicates his toilet needs occasionally.* She *lets him carry breakables* such as glasses and dishes. He *helps to put things away* and *pushes a large toy with good steering,* backing out of corners by himself.

EXAMINATION SEQUENCE

Locomotor (Child's Table and Chair)

21–24 Months   *Situation No.**
Table and Chair
Picture Book 46
Cubes: Tower 12
       Train 13
       Chimney 14
Cup and Cubes 17
Pegboard 27
Safety Pin 29
Body Parts 47
Drawing: Spontaneous 34
       Vertical Stroke 36
       Circular Scribble 37
       Horizontal Stroke 38
Picture Cards 48
Formboard 42
Vertical Slot or Performance Box 43
Color Forms 44
Toy and Stick 28
Test Objects 52
Small Ball: Ball Play 58
       Directions 59
       In Basket or Performance Box 60
Large Ball 69
Walking, Running 70
Jumping 73
Standing 72
Stairs 71

Italicized items appear for the first time in this sequence.
*Situation number identifies the examination situation described in Chapter 4, Examination Procedures.

H = **History**
O = **Observation**
(*) = **Pattern replaced by more mature one at later age.**

H	O	21 Months
		ADAPTIVE
		Cubes: tower of 6 Cubes: aligns 3 for train Toy & Stick: tries to get toy, no demonstration (*24m) Formboard: adapts to rotation, corrects error (*30m) Vertical Slot: inserts square, no demonstration Basket or Box: retrieves ball, tips or crawls in
		GROSS MOTOR
		Walks: runs well Stairs: walks up, holds rail Stairs: walks down, holds rail Large Ball: kicks, demonstration (*24m)
		FINE MOTOR
		Cubes: tower of 6
		LANGUAGE
		Vocabulary: 30–50 words Speech: uses "me" Speech: uses "mine" Picture Book: names 1 Picture Card: names 1 Test Objects: names 3 Picture Book: points to 3 Picture Card: points to 4 Test Objects: points to 4 Body Parts: points to 6 Ball: follows 4 directional commands
		PERSONAL-SOCIAL
		Feeding: bottle discarded Feeding: eats with fork Play: hands cup full of cubes Play: pretends to feed, dress doll or animal Dress: unzips own zippers Mirror: identifies self (*30m)

H	O	KEY AGE: 24 Months
		ADAPTIVE
		Cubes: tower of 7 Cubes: aligns 4 for train Draw: imitates vertical stroke (*36m) Draw: imitates circular scribble (*30m) Toy & Stick: gets toy, no demonstration Formboard: inserts 3 blocks spontaneously Color Forms: places 2
		GROSS MOTOR
		Jumps: both feet off floor Jumps: from bottom step both feet at once Stands: tries on 1 foot without holding Large Ball: kicks on request
		FINE MOTOR
		Cubes: tower of 7 Safety Pin: threads shoelace through Pegboard: inserts large square immediately Pegboard: inserts small square immediately
		LANGUAGE
		Vocabulary: 50+ words Speech: uses "I" Speech: uses "you" Speech: jargon discarded Speech: 3- or 4-word sentences Speech: uses plurals Speech: rhymes, songs—fills in words (*36m) Picture Book: names 2 Picture Card: names 3 Test Objects: names 4 Body Parts: names at least 1 Picture Book: identifies action (*30m) Picture Cards: points to 7 Body Parts: points to 7
		PERSONAL-SOCIAL
		Feeding: feeds self, spills little Toilet: occasionally indicates needs (*36m) Communication: verbalizes immediate experiences Communication: refers to self by pronoun Play: pushes toy with good steering Play: helps put things away Play: carries breakables

GLOSSARY

21 Months

ADAPTIVE

Cubes: tower of 6. Successfully stacks 6 blocks; tower falls with 7th. (See 24 months.)

Cubes: aligns 3 for train. Child imitates horizontal combination of at least 3 cubes, after examiner demonstrates and then dismantles train.

Toy and Stick: tries to get toy, no demonstration. Child uses stick to try to get toy on request, but does not succeed.

Formboard: adapts to rotation, corrects error. Child makes mistakes, but corrects them with each rotation, Examiner tells child to look at all the holes but does not point to correct ones.

Vertical Slot or Performance Box: inserts square, no demonstration. Spontaneously adapts block completely to hole.

Basket or Performance Box: retrieves ball, tips or crawls in. Any method such as pushing box over, lifting and tilting box, creeping into box after overturning it. Repeat if performance seems highly accidental. Situation cannot be used with children tall enough to reach ball. This is an excellent situation in which to observe reactions of the child in face of difficulties—persistence, ingenuity, emotional responses, etc.

GROSS MOTOR

Walks: runs well. Knees flex and arms alternate fairly well and balance maintained, but still does not go very fast. Stops without having to reach some barrier.

Stairs: walks up, holds rail. Both feet brought to each step in succession. Erect position.

Stairs: walks down, holds rail. See definition above.

Large Ball: kicks, demonstration. Without holding on for support, child swings leg and strikes ball. (See 24 months.)

FINE MOTOR

Cubes: tower of 6. Tower stands without assistance from examiner.

LANGUAGE

Vocabulary: 30–50 words. May be understood only by family members, but articulation improving.

Speech: uses "me." Usually used correctly in referring to self.

Speech: uses "mine." Usually used correctly.

Picture Book: names 1. Dog, baby, shoe, etc.

Picture Card: names 1. Usually dog or shoe. (See 24 months.)

Test Objects: names 3. On request. (See 24 months.)

Picture Book: identifies 3. Child points, or if shy or wary, clearly looks at. Total includes those already named correctly.

Picture Card: points to 4. Total includes those already named correctly.

Test Objects: points to 4. Total includes those already named correctly.

Body Parts: points to 6. Total includes those already named correctly. (See 24 months.)

Ball: follows 4 directional commands. Complies on verbal request only. May throw ball at chair, table, mother or examiner, but not seat self on chair holding ball.

PERSONAL–SOCIAL

Feeding: bottle discarded. Takes milk and other liquids *entirely* from cup or glass.

Feeding: eats with fork. Eats part of meal with a fork, using fork to get food, not simply using hands to put food on fork.

Play: hands cup full of cubes. At completion of Cubes Situations, fills cup and hands it to examiner, spontaneously or on request. Younger child starts taking cubes out one by one or dumps them all.

Play: pretends to feed, dress, doll or animal. Self-explanatory.

Dressing: unzips own zippers. Zippers on another person or large zippers on play objects easier to manipulate.

Mirror: identifies self. Child definitely points to image of self on request.

24 Months

ADAPTIVE

Cubes: tower of 7. Successfully stacks 7 cubes; tower falls with 8th. May need demonstration to begin and urging to continue. Examiner may assist with holding if child with motor abnormality indicates intent to build by bringing successive cubes to tower.

Cubes: aligns 4 for train. Child imitates horizontal combination of all 4 cubes after examiner demonstrates and then dismantles train.

Drawing: imitates vertical stroke. Makes definite stroke with correct directional orientation. (See 36 months.)

Drawing: imitates circular scribble. Differentiates clearly from vertical stroke and makes series of circles on top of each other. (See 30 months.)

Formboard: inserts 3 spontaneously. Inserts blocks completely into correct holes, spontaneously or on request, without any adjusting by examiner.

Color Forms: places 2. Child must place 2 additional forms correctly if round form needs to be demonstrated.

Toy and Stick: gets toy, no demonstration. Child uses stick to get toy on request.

GROSS MOTOR

Jumps: both feet off floor. Both feet off floor simultaneously, in place, after demonstration.

Jumps: from bottom step, both feet at once. Jumps, not walks, off. Lands erect.

Stands: tries on 1 foot without holding. Examiner demonstrates, maintaining pose to encourage child to do so. Holding on for support not permitted.

Large Ball: kicks on request. Child swings leg to strike ball, without holding on for support. (See 21 months.)

FINE MOTOR

Cubes: tower of 7. Tower stands without assistance from examiner.

Safety Pin: threads shoelace through. Child threads end of shoelace through hole at closed end of safety pin after demonstration.

Pegboard: inserts large square immediately. Indicates awareness of how peg goes in and inserts large square smoothly on first or second attempt.

Pegboard: inserts small square immediately. See above definition.

LANGUAGE

Vocabulary: 50+ words. Too many to count. Articulation relatively clear, but may not be.

Speech: uses "I." Usually used correctly.

Speech: uses "you." Usually used correctly.

Speech: jargon discarded. Words may not be well-articulated, but clearly are meant to be words, not merely sounds with inflections. (See 52 weeks.)

Speech: 3- or 4-word sentences. Caution is necessary in accepting such sentences as "I don't know," or "I love you," if they are only ones used by child.

Speech: uses plurals. Says "dogs, babies, shoes," etc., if there are more than one.

Speech: rhymes, songs—fills in words. Supplies missing words at beginning or end of rhyme or song but cannot get all the way through by self.

Picture Book: names 2. On request.

Picture Card: names 3. On request. Dog (or any animal), shoe, cup (container, *not* contents), house. (See 36 months.)

Test Objects: names 4. Pencil, key, penny, shoe, ball.

Body Parts: names at least 1. On doll, child's own body, mother's or examiner's body.

Picture Book: identifies action. Points to correct picture as examiner asks for baby sleeping, eating, etc.

Picture Card: points to 7. Total includes those already named correctly.

Body Parts: points to all 7. Total includes those already named correctly.

PERSONAL–SOCIAL

Feeding: feeds self, spills little. Feeds self neatly with spoon without help.

Toilet: occasionally indicates needs. Sometimes lets mother know ahead of time, both bowel and urine control.

Communication: verbalizes immediate experiences. Talks about activities as they are occurring, *e.g.*, "I read book," "Me ride wagon."

Communication: refers to self by pronoun. Calls self by "I" or "me" rather than by own name.

Play: pushes toy with good steering. Wagon, doll carriage or other large vehicle; backs out of corners without help.

Play: helps put things away. Assists on request from mother with toys, dishes, etc.

Play: carries breakables. Mother allows child to carry glasses, dishes, ash trays, etc.

36 MONTHS

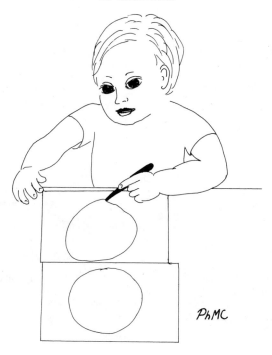

Copies circle, holds crayon by fingers

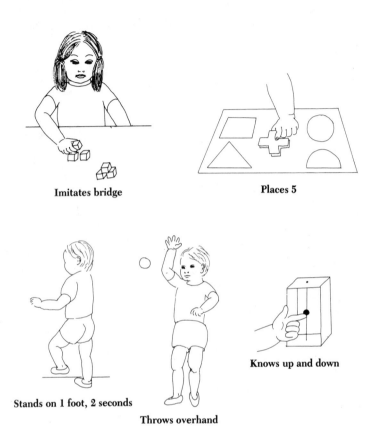

Imitates bridge

Places 5

Stands on 1 foot, 2 seconds

Throws overhand

Knows up and down

The 3-year-old accepts a chair readily and, depending upon her social environment and conditioning, remains seated and responds appropriately as long as the examination requires. She turns the pages of the PICTURE BOOK singly, names the pictures, and tells the action delineated, *e.g.*, the baby is sleeping.

The CUBES are presented and the "house" or TOWER is requested. The child builds a *tower of ten cubes*. On demonstration of the TRAIN, four cubes with a fifth superimposed as a CHIMNEY, she duplicates it. The examiner builds a three-cube BRIDGE out of the child's sight, then points to the component parts and hands her three more cubes. If she is unable to copy the bridge, the examiner demonstrates its construction with running comment. The child *imitates the bridge* accurately.

The BOTTLE AND TEN PELLETS are placed before the child, in a position which favors the use of the child's preferred hand, and she is asked to put them all in the bottle, one at a time, just as fast as she can. She *puts in all ten sequentially in 25 seconds or less* in the best of two or three trials.

The BEADS are dumped out of the tube onto the table and the child is asked to put them back. She holds the tube with one hand and inserts the beads with the other.

The examiner shows the child a doll and asks her to name the eyes, nose, mouth, etc. She names seven BODY PARTS.

Given a paper and crayon for DRAWING, she *holds the crayon with her fingers,* adult fashion. She scribbles and, in response to a question, "NAMES" what she has drawn. She *copies the* VERTICAL *and* HORIZONTAL STROKES *and a CIRCLE from models. She imitates the* CROSS the examiner has drawn, but may use four separate strokes instead of two crossed lines. She names the INCOMPLETE MAN but in response to the questions, "What does he need?" "What's missing?," she scribbles indiscriminately, even when specific parts lacking are pointed out.

She *tries to cut with* SCISSORS, opening the blades, although she usually is not successful.

The examiner shows the PICTURE CARDS and asks the child to name each picture in turn. She *names all ten* pictures correctly.

The FORMBOARD is presented with each block in front of its appropriate hole. She inserts the blocks in their correct holes immediately and responds to the 180° rotation of the board by adapting to the reversal without error or with immediate correction of her error.

The placard carrying the five red COLOR FORMS is placed on the table and the child is asked to place the circle, square, triangle, semicircle and cross, one after the other. She *places all five forms* without demonstration.

She then is given the card with the ten black and white GEOMETRIC FORMS from the Stanford-Binet test. She is handed the small cards one at a time and asked to place the forms where they fit. The circle may be demonstrated. She *points to or places seven* forms correctly.

On request she *gives her full* NAME and *tells her* SEX in response to the question, "Are you a little girl or a little boy?"

She is asked three simple COMPREHENSION A QUESTIONS, "What do you do when you are hungry? . . . sleepy? . . . cold?" She *answers one* question satisfactorily.

Her immediate recall is tested by asking her to repeat the DIGITS 4–2, 6–3, 5–8, then 6–4–1, 3–5–2, and 8–3–7. She *repeats one set of three* digits correctly.

Her understanding of a series of CONCEPTS is evaluated. She is given the BIG and LITTLE blocks of similar color and asked to hand the examiner the big one. She gives the large one consistently on three trials. Alternatively, she may hand the big one and name the little one on the first trial.

The examiner brings out the box and shows the child how to move the bead UP AND DOWN on the string. The child *indicates her awarness* of the concept by moving the bead consistently in the correct direction.

The examiner presents the LOUD AND SOFT noise containers, shaking first one and then the other. The child *gives the container requested* correctly on three trials. Alternatively, she may name the sound of the remaining container after having handed one correctly.

If the child succeeds in these three situations, she is given the LIGHTEST and HEAVIEST of the five weighted blocks, one for each hand, and is asked to give the examiner the heavy block. Only rarely is she able to give the heaviest block in two of three trials.

Introducing the ACTION AGENT situation the examiner asks, "What runs? . . . What cries?" If the child does not respond, the examiner answers for her and proceeds with the rest of the questions (flies, bites, sleeps, scratches, swims, cuts, burns, blows, etc.) The child *answers* with the subject of the verb for *four* of the words.

The four small colored blocks are presented and the child asked to name red, yellow, green and blue in turn. If she does not do so, she is asked to identify the COLORS and she *points to two* of the four blocks correctly.

She names all of the TEST OBJECTS (pencil, key, penny, examiner's shoe) and *gives the* USE *of two* of them.

She then is given the SMALL BALL and the table is moved to one side so that she may stand and walk about. She THROWS *the ball overhand* and then *carries out three of* the following PREPOSI-TIONAL directions: "Put the ball on, under, in front of, in back of and beside the chair."

She kicks the LARGE BALL with facility, *does a broad jump*, using both feet at once, and STANDS *on one foot for two seconds* without holding on, in imitation of the examiner. She is reported to ride a tricycle, steering and using the pedals. She *alternates her feet* going up and *down* STAIRS in adult fashion.

Her vocabulary contains innumerable words and she speaks in

well-formed eight- or nine-word sentences and *puts sentences together with "and" and "but."* She carries a recognizable tune and *recites TV commercials, rhymes, or songs all the way through.* She *understands taking turns* and is reported to play with other children in *associative play.* She *takes care of her own toilet needs* and *generally is dry at night.* Her mother reports that she also *knows the front from the back* of her clothes and *dresses herself with some supervision.* She can be trusted to *wash and dry her hands,* not just play in the water.

EXAMINATION SEQUENCE
Locomotor (Child's Table and Chair)

30–36 Months	Situation No.*
Table and Chair	
Picture Book	46
Cubes: Tower	12
Train	13
Chimney	14
Bridge	15
10 Pellets and Bottle	23
Beads	30
Body Parts	47
Drawing: Spontaneous	34
Vertical Stroke	36
Horizontal Stroke	38
Circle	39
Cross	40
Incomplete Man	41
Scissors	31
Picture Cards	48
Formboard	42
Color Forms	44
Geometric Forms	45
Name and Sex	49
Comprehension A Questions	50
Digits	51
Concepts: Big and Little	55
Up and Down	56
Loud and Soft	57
Action Agents	53
Colors	54
Test Objects	52
Small Ball: Ball Play	58
Prepositions	61
Large Ball	69
Postural: Jumping	73
Standing	72
Stairs	71

Italicized items appear for the first time in this sequence
*Situation number identifies the examination situation described in Chapter 4, Examination Procedures.

H = **History**
O = **Observation**
(*) = **Pattern replaced by more mature one at later age.**

H	O	30 Months
		ADAPTIVE
		Cubes: tower of 9 Cubes: adds chimney to train Pellets & Bottle: pellets in, 1 at a time Beads: inserts into tube Draw: names own drawing Draw: imitates horizontal stroke (*36m) Draw: imitates circle (*36m) Draw: 2 or more strokes for cross (*36m) Draw: names incomplete man Formboard: adapts to rotation immediately Color Forms: places 4 Digits: repeats 2, 1 of 3 trials
		GROSS MOTOR
		Stairs: alternates feet going up Rides: tricycle, using pedals Stands: 1 foot, momentary balance
		FINE MOTOR
		Cubes: tower of 9 Picture Book: turns pages singly Pellets: in bottle, 30 seconds or less
		LANGUAGE
		Speech: 8- or 9-word sentences Speech: carries recognizable tune Communication: uses "he" and "she" correctly Communication: relates events of 2–3 days ago Picture Book: gives action Picture Cards: names 8 Test Objects: gives use of 1 Body Parts: names 7 Picture Cards: points to all Test Objects: indicates use of key or penny Concepts: knows big & little Prepositions: follows 2 commands
		PERSONAL-SOCIAL
		Feeding: pours well from glass to glass Play: keeps time to music by stamping, clapping Dress: pulls up pants Dress: finds armholes correctly Dress: puts on shoes, any foot (*42m) Mirror: names mirror image

H	O	KEY AGE: 36 Months
		ADAPTIVE
		Cubes: tower of 10 Cubes: imitates bridge (*42m) Draw: copies vertical stroke Draw: copies horizontal stroke Draw: copies circle Draw: imitates cross (*——) Color Forms: places 5 Geometric Forms: places 7 Digits: repeats 3, 1 of 3 trials
		GROSS MOTOR
		Stairs: alternates feet going down Jumps: broad jump Stands: on 1 foot, 2 seconds Ball: throws overhand
		FINE MOTOR
		Cubes: tower of 10 Pellets: in bottle, 25 seconds or less Draw: holds crayon by fingers Scissors: tries to cut (*——)
		LANGUAGE
		Speech: puts sentence together with "and" or "but" Communication: recites all of rhymes, songs Picture Card: names all Test Objects: gives use of 2 Name: gives full name Sex: tells sex Action Agent: gives 4 Comprehension A: answers 1 question Concepts: knows up & down Concepts: knows loud & soft Colors: identifies 2 (*42m) Prepositions: follows 3 commands
		PERSONAL-SOCIAL
		Toilet: goes alone, dry at night Communication: understands taking turns Play: associative play (*——) Dress: washes, dries hands Dress: dresses with supervision (*——) Dress: knows front from back

GLOSSARY

30 Months

ADAPTIVE

Cubes: tower of 9. (See 36 months.)

Cubes: adds chimney to train. Examiner may ask where chimney is if child responds to demonstration and dismantling of model only by aligning cubes.

Pellet and Bottle: pellets in, one at a time. Child may pick up more than one pellet at a time, provided they are dropped in singly. Examiner may need to continue urging, "One at a time."

Beads: inserts into tube. Child must hold tube in one hand and beads in other to succeed in activity. Indicates awareness that beads must go in singly, rather than trying to stuff in by whole handfuls. Examiner may demonstrate after unsuccessful attempts.

Drawing: names own drawing. Spontaneously or on request, although only a scribble is made. Child's verbalization does not have to be adult word.

Drawing: imitates horizontal stroke. Correct directional orientation and usually only single imitative stroke. (See 36 months.)

Drawing: imitates circle. Differentiates clearly from strokes, and may make more than single large circle. (See 36 months.)

Drawing: 2 or more strokes for cross. Imitates by more than 1 stroke, without correct orientation. Performance should be different from child's response to stroke demonstration. (See 36 months.)

Drawing: names incomplete man. "Snowman," or any response indicating person.

Formboard: adapts to rotation immediately. Makes no error or corrects own error immediately.

Color Forms: places 4. Child must place rest of forms correctly if round form needs to be demonstrated.

Digits: repeats 2, 1 of 3 trials. Repeats in correct order after examiner has finished pair.

GROSS MOTOR

Stairs: alternates feet going up. In adult fashion, 1 foot to each step.

Rides: tricycle, using pedals. Propels and steers without assistance.

Stands: 1 foot, momentary balance. Manages to hold foot up. (See 36 months.)

FINE MOTOR

Cubes: tower of 9. Tower stands without assistance from examiner.

Picture Book: turns pages singly. Distinguish intent to turn pages one at a time from accidental occurrence.

Pellets: in bottle, 30 seconds or less. Must be put in one at a time.

LANGUAGE

Speech: 8- or 9-word sentences. Self-explanatory.

Speech: carries recognizable tune. What child is trying to produce can be discerned clearly.

Communication: uses "he" and "she" correctly. Usually used in referring to playmates, siblings, etc.

Communication: relates events of 2 or 3 days ago. Self-explanatory.

Picture Book: gives action. Describes baby sleeping, eating, etc.

Picture Cards: names 8. On request. (See 24 and 36 months.)

Test Objects: gives use of 1. Tells what is done with object. (See 36 months.)

Body Parts: names 7. On doll, own body, mother's or examiner's body.

Picture Cards: points to all. Total includes those already named correctly.

Test Objects: indicates use of key or penny. Takes key to or holds it out towards door, makes sound of car running, puts penny in pocket, etc. Obviously understands use if has verbalized it already.

Concepts: knows big and little. Hands block asked for consistently.

Prepositions: follows 2 commands. On verbal request only. (See 36 months.)

PERSONAL–SOCIAL

Feeding: pours well from glass to glass. Judges quantity correctly, without much spilling. May even pour from pitcher.

Play: keeps time to music by stamping, clapping. Not necessarily the correct beat, but child shows definite attempts at rhythm.

Dressing: pulls up pants. After mother has started child finishes job, pulling completely up.

Dressing: finds armholes correctly. Puts on jacket, coat, cardigan completely, without any assistance.

Dressing: puts on shoes, any foot. Manages to get *shoes* on, though not necessarily on correct feet.

Mirror: names mirror image. Says "me" or gives name.

36 Months

ADAPTIVE

Cubes: tower of 10. Successfully stacks all cubes. May need demonstration to begin and urging to continue. Examiner may assist with holding if child indicates intent to build by bringing successive cubes to tower, but has a motor disability.

Cubes: imitates bridge. Places cubes correctly, with top cube bridging space between 2 base cubes.

Drawing: copies vertical stroke. Reproduces correct directional orientation from model on card. (See 24 months.)

Drawing: copies horizontal stroke. See above definition. (See 30 months.)

Drawing: copies circle. Reproduces model on card. May make more than single circle. (See 30 months.)

Drawing: imitates cross. Essential feature is recognition of different orientation of two lines. May be produced in three or four segments rather than by 2 strokes. (See 30 months.)

Color Forms: places 5. All forms placed correctly on request.

Geometric Forms: places 7. Child places 7 more correctly if round form needs to be demonstrated.

Digits: repeats 3, 1 of 3 trials. Repeats in correct order after examiner has finished a set.

GROSS MOTOR

Stairs: alternates feet going down. Adult fashion, bringing 1 foot to each step.

Jumps: broad jump. With *both* feet at *same time*, covering distance.

Stands: on 1 foot, 2 seconds. Examiner demonstrates, maintains pose and counts out loud to encourage child. Holding on for support not permitted.

Ball: throws overhand. Definitely raises arm to shoulder height or above and pronates to throw.

FINE MOTOR

Cubes: tower of 10. Tower stands without assistance from examiner.

Pellets: in bottle, 25 seconds or less. Pellets must be inserted singly.

Drawing: holds crayon by fingers. Adult fashion, as opposed to using fist.

Scissors: tries to cut. Gets blades to move up and down but does not necessarily succeed in cutting.

LANGUAGE

Speech: puts sentences together with "and" or "but." Self-explanatory.

Communication: recites all of rhymes, songs. Gets all the way through rhymes or songs correctly rather than just filling in words. (See 24 months.)

Picture Card: names all. On request. Clock, basket (pocketbook), book, flag, leaf (tree, flower), star. (See 24 months.)

Test Objects: gives use of 2. Tells what is done with objects. Pencil, key, penny (put in pocket, gum, candy, etc.).

Name: gives full name. Nickname permitted for first name.

Sex: tells sex. Gives own sex correctly.

Action Agent: gives 4. Gives subject, not object, of verb. "Fire burns," not "Burns me."

Comprehension A: answers 1 question. Single-word answers of appropriate nouns or verbs acceptable.

Concepts: knows up and down. Moves bead in correct direction consistently.

Concepts: knows loud and soft. Gives correct container consistently.

Colors: identifies 2. Total includes those already named correctly, if any.

Prepositions: follows 3 commands. On verbal request only. On, under, in back of, in front of, beside. Obeying only "on the chair" indicates knowing chair, not preposition.

PERSONAL–SOCIAL

Toilet: goes alone, dry at night. Child fully toilet trained.

Communication: understands taking turns. Waits while other child or adult takes turn.

Play: associative play. Several children engage in same activity, with frequent cross-references common. Child playing *with* other children, not merely alongside them doing what they are doing.

Dressing: washes, dries hands. Child completes job without playing in water when mother sends child in to clean up.

Dressing: dresses with supervision. Child gets most of clothes on by self if mother has laid clothes out and assists with small parts or hard to reach items.

Dressing: knows front from back. Has no difficulty with items which have clearly distinguishable fronts and backs.

4
Examination Techniques

INTRODUCTION TO THE EXAMINATION

Preliminaries and introductory procedures must be adapted to the general maturity characteristics of the child. Before the interview begins, the appropriate forms should be collated, and the examining equipment and materials positioned properly for the expected behavior the child will exhibit. Special suggestions and directions for making an easy, natural transition to the formal examination are given briefly below.

Note that the mother takes the active part in the introductory procedures. The examiner does not touch the child, but keeps at a distance. This applies to all the age ranges. The mother removes shoes and stockings from an *infant* during the interview; other clothing is removed prior to the postural situations unless it interferes with the examination before this.

4–20 Weeks Maturity. At a favorable moment when the infant is quiet and contented, ask the mother to place him on his back on the crib platform or examining table. The examiner stands at the infant's left; the mother is invited to take a chair placed at the infant's right when it is clear that the infant is happy. The Supine situations follow. Many 16- and 20-week olds may resent the supine position; the mother should be asked if her infant prefers the sitting position.

24–32 Weeks Maturity. At a favorable moment while you are interviewing the mother, when the infant is unapprehensive and playful, offer her an introductory toy, such as the tricolored rings or catbells. When she accepts it, she has accepted you. If she is empty-handed when it is time to proceed to the examination, and especially if a transition from another room has been made, reoffer a toy. When she accepts it, place a second introductory toy on the table in plain view, and take your place at the left of the crib or examining table. If a clinical crib and chair are available, ask the mother, who is on the right of the crib, to place the infant in the chair and to "stand by" until all is well. The belt has been attached on the mother's side of the chair, left unfastened on the examiner's side. Secure the belt tightly around her chest; the infant is better able to tolerate what appears to be excessive compression than any degree of looseness which permits her to slump. Insufficient chest support interferes with adequate arm control. Move the tabletop into position, and if necessary, call the infant's attention to the toy on the table. As soon as she begins to play, the mother sits down at the right. If there is no crib, the infant examining chair and portable test table are utilized, on any available flat surface. If there is no special clinical examining equipment available, ask the mother to seat herself in a chair at a desk and hold the infant on her lap. The mother supports the infant *firmly* around the chest with both hands, leaving both of the child's arms free for exploitation. The appropriate Tabletop situations follow.

36–52 Weeks Maturity. Offer the introductory toy as for the 24–32 week maturity levels; when the infant accepts it, ask the mother to place him seated on the crib platform or examining table before the tabletop. She stands by until all is well. The tabletop is moved into place by the examiner, who stands at the left (the mother again is at the right), and the infant's attention is called to the introductory toy on the tabletop. As soon as the infant begins to play, the mother sits down. The appropriate Tabletop situations follow.

56 Weeks–15 Months Maturity. At this age the size of the child is the chief factor in determining where the examination is done. If she is physically large, then placement in the kindergarten chair before the kindergarten table probably is best (see 18–36 Months, below). If she is small, then the examination is conducted best at the adjustable clinical table used for the interview, with the child on the mother's lap. The bag of varicolored building blocks which was on the table when mother and child entered the room, and with which the child was playing during the interview, is removed and is replaced by the Picture Book, which the examiner begins to demonstrate.

18–36 Months Maturity. The child is invited to play with some toys. He is shown the kindergarten table with a bag of varicolored blocks on it, and shown his chair. The mother seats herself at the right of the table, the examiner at the left. The mother may be asked to help the child into his chair. When the interview is over, the child is asked to help put the blocks back into the bag because there are more toys to play with. This task is completed, with or without the child's cooperation, and when the child is in position behind the table, seated or perhaps still standing, the examiner begins to demonstrate the Picture Book which follows.

Modifications for Special Circumstances. If the infant is emotionally fragile, cries and is unwilling to leave her mother, the examination is carried out at the adjustable clinical table with her on her mother's lap. Usually, by the time the postural situations are reached, the infant is sufficiently disarmed to accept placement in the crib; the mother keeps her hands on her and cuddles close when she first places her before the mirror. The examiner will have to decide in each instance whether or not to risk trying the examination in the crib first, and should not hesitate to return the infant to the mother's lap if necessary. A fragile older child also may need to start out on the mother's lap.

The best dictum when the child is suspicious is, *"Examiner, withdraw."* Sit back in your chair and increase the distance between yourself and the child. If the child is inhibited and won't participate, let the mother offer the test object at the beginning. If that fails, put one on the tabletop, pick up a book or papers, hand a book to mother, and ignore him. It may take 15–30 minutes and changes of the items offered, with occasional comments and demonstrations, before the child breaks through and participates. With an older child, the formboard often is successful as a last resort; with an infant, the bell.

If the child has a motor handicap for which she needs assistance with sitting, she is strapped into the supporting chair or held on her mother's lap, depending on her age and size, but the initial sequence may be the one appropriate to her chronologic rather than her motor age. (See Chapter 10 of *Developmental Diagnosis.*)

EXAMINATION SEQUENCES

So far as possible, the standard sequences should be followed in the administration of the examination situations. The standard sequence differs with the maturity and age of the child. There are 3 maturity zones: Supine; sitting, either with support or free; and locomotor. The recommended standard sequence for each of these maturity zones accompanies the Developmental Schedule for the appropriate Key Age.

EXAMINATION PROCEDURES

The purpose of this section is to outline in detail the procedures used in administering the individual situations. The general character of these procedures already has been indicated in Chapter 3. The procedures described here are appropriate for children at the stated ages or maturity levels. For deviant children with motor or sensory handicaps, modifications may be necessary; these in turn will need to be interpreted in light of the clinical nature of the abnormality.

Although the situations are discussed separately here, the examiner should not regard them as a series of rigidly separate tests. The examination should be conducted as an organic unit; the transition from one situation to the next should be accomplished in such a way that the child's working rapport is not only preserved but actually increased. The examiner should shift readily to a higher or lower maturity level when the child's performance indicates a change is necessary. On the other hand, the examination must not assume so much informality that the situations lose their integrity as diagnostic tools. They should be administered in the prescribed standardized manner. The examiner must strike a very careful balance between uniformity and variation.

For each situation, an opportunity for exhibiting the most advanced behavior should always be given, *i.e.*, asking the child to name before pointing, the examiner using request and gesture before demonstration. Making a verbal request and pointing to induce performance is not the same as demonstrating, and should be the first approach. Actual demonstration of the performance follows if there is no response. The child's attention should be secured to all demonstrations. The examiner is not trying to trick the child. *Never* give the child a chance to refuse by asking, "Do you want to. . . ," Would you like to. . . ." *Always* phrase activities positively: "We are going to. . . ," etc.

The examiner must maintain firm control of the situation at all times and may have to ask the parent to desist from interfering. It goes without saying that he treats the child and the parents with courtesy, indicates his approval of the child's behavior and, of course, says "please" and "thank you."

In the following syllabus, each situation carries an identification number in the left margin; these assigned numbers are referred to in the examination sequence which accompanies each Key Age Developmental Schedule in Chapter 3.

SUPINE SITUATIONS

1. Supine

4–20 Weeks Maturity. The examiner simply observes the infant's posture and spontaneous activity. If necessary, he may be spoken to in a reassuring tone.

At *24 weeks* the infant may resent being placed down, and the supine situation follows all other situations. Offer the dangling ring or rattle immediately without preliminary observation. If the infant is not appeased immediately, terminate the examination.

2. Dangling Ring

4–20 Weeks Maturity. The end of the string is held in the examiner's left hand, and the ring permitted to hang down. In this manner the ring is brought about 4–6 inches above the infant's feet and then moved headward. The ring is held 10–12 inches above the face. If the infant's head remains turned to the side, move the ring into the line of vision. Observe the reaction to the perception of the ring.

4–16 Weeks Maturity: Ring-Following. Move the ring slowly through an arc of 180° from one side of the infant's head to the other, keeping the distance from the head about constant. If regard shifts to the examiner's hand, continue the arc until the hand rests on the crib platform. After side-to-side following, the dangled ring is moved vertically, beginning at the infant's eye level. It is moved slowly from a position above the head to a position above the chest. Circular following is elicited by moving the dangled ring in a slow circular motion around the face. Repeated trials may be made, and every opportunity should be given the infant to demonstrate the optimal capacity to follow a moving object (ring or examiner's hand). The speed of the moving ring should be adapted to the infant's abilities in ocular pursuit.

12–20 Weeks Maturity: Ring Exploitation. If the infant reaches for the ring immediately, ring-following is omitted. The ring is held suspended within reach above the upper chest, and the infant's prehensory efforts are observed. The ring may be steadied if it is set swinging. If it is not grasped, it is then held about 1 inch from the *palm* to see if this distance can be completed. If necessary it is placed in the hand; the hand most favorable for ring regard is selected first. The perceptual and manipulatory exploitation of the ring is observed. Both hands are tried and any difference in control noted. If the ring drops before observations are complete, it may be restored to the hand; otherwise it is recovered gently and the Rattle situation (3) presented immediately. If regard for the examiner predominates, she steps out of range of the infant's vision. If tonic-neck-reflex positions persist after 12 weeks and interfere with exploitation, the examiner gently cradles the infant's head in her palm to assist in maintaining midpositions, at the same time allowing free head rotation. This technique permits distinguishing motor from adaptive components of behavior.

3. Rattle

4–24 Weeks Maturity. The rattle is held in the examiner's left hand, presented *silently* over the infant's feet and moved to within reaching distance over the upper chest of the supine infant. The perceptual response is observed; the rattle may be moved into the line of vision if the infant's head is averted, or it may be shaken gently to elicit attention. After side-to-side following, the rattle is moved vertically, beginning at the infant's eye level. It is moved slowly from a position above the head to a position above the chest. Circular following is elicited by moving the rattle in a slow circular motion around the face. The infant is allowed to grasp the handle of the rattle if possible, or it is brought near the hand, or finally placed in the hand. The hand most favorable for rattle regard is selected first, and the fingers may have to be opened. Exploitation of the rattle is observed and also the response to loss of the rattle. If it is retained, it is removed gently while the infant is looking at it and placed to the side within the visual field to determine the infant's ability to look after and pursue the lost rattle and to roll to the prone position.

4. Social Stimulation

4–24 Weeks Maturity. The infant is shifted gently to lie across the table or crib; the examiner may make the shift himself, taking his position at the infant's feet. The examiner bends over the infant and smiles, talks and nods his head, endeavoring to elicit attention and social response. The situation is not prolonged; it is continuous with the Bird Call, Bell-Ringing situation (5). After *24 Weeks,* social responses are elicited opportunistically.

5. Bird Call, Bell-Ringing

4–24 Weeks Maturity. While the infant is active and the examiner is talking, the bird call is twisted gently two or three times. It is held 2-3 inches from first one ear and then the other, and the infant's responses are noted. If there is no response, the bell then is rung fairly sharply in a similar manner. The examiner should take care that the infant does not spy the examiner's hand or the objects. If the infant is exploiting a toy and makes no response, the toy should be removed before the procedure is repeated. If the infant objects to the supine position, the behavior should be elicited with the infant in the sitting position. Between *28* and *52 weeks* it is elicited while the infant is sitting. In older children if there is any question of hearing defect, this behavior should be elicited opportunistically.

6. Pull-to-Sitting

4–24 Weeks Maturity. Having secured the infant's attention, the examiner holds the infant's hands in her own and exerts gentle, steady forward traction on the arms. If the infant's head lags excessively, the traction is released and the infant raised to the sitting position with head supported. Otherwise, the pull-to-sitting is completed, and the infant's head control and participation in the pull are noted.

TABLETOP SITUATIONS

Between *12 and 20 weeks,* the tabletop situations follow the Pull-to-Sitting situation (6). At *24 weeks* of age and thereafter, the examination begins with the tabletop situations. At *24 weeks*, the supine situations follow the tabletop and postural situations. Thereafter, the supine situations are omitted.

Presentation. From *12–56 weeks,* a standard procedure is used to present all single test objects of this group. Each object, held in the examiner's left hand, is brought to the center of the far edge of the table; the infant's attention to the presentation is elicited, by tapping the object against the table edge if necessary. In extreme cases it may be necessary to use other methods to elicit attention; their use should be noted. When attention is secured, the object is brought *smoothly* toward the infant and placed within easy reach on the table. The object should be held so that it is more conspicuous than the examiner's hand. Placement should be central to favor a free choice of handedness in grasp. The examiner should withdraw his hand as inconspicuously as possible.

From *15 to 36 months,* the presentations are made by simply reaching in from the left and placing the test objects within easy reach on the table before the child. The presentation of multiple object situations will be described individually.

Transitions. In making the transition from one situation to another in the tabletop situations, the examiner should take advantage of the infant's dropping a toy to subsitute the next. If it is necessary to remove a toy from the infant's hand, it should be grasped lightly, and then the examiner should wait until the infant releases the object. At times it is necessary, when presenting the next object, to permit the infant to retain the one in hand until it can be withdrawn opportunistically. Transitions should be made smoothly, and *the infant should never have to wait* for the next object.

No situation is prolonged. One or two minutes of exploitation usually is ample, but sometimes two or three demonstrations are necessary before the child performs.

7. First Cube

12–56 Weeks Maturity. The cube is presented and the infant's responses observed. Before *24 weeks* of age, the cube is offered to his hand or even placed in the hand, after initial responses are observed.

8. Second Cube

16–56 Weeks Maturity. While the infant is holding the 1st cube, a 2nd is presented in a similar manner and the response is observed. Before *24 weeks* of age, it may be placed in his hand after initial responses are observed.

9. Third Cube

20–56 Weeks Maturity. While the infant is holding 2 cubes, the 3rd cube is presented and the response observed. Before *24 weeks* of age, the cubes may be placed in the hands after initial responses are observed, or contact and grasp maintained by placing the infant's hands on top of the cubes on the table.

10. Tower of Two

48–56 Weeks Maturity. The examiner secures the child's attention, then builds a tower of only 2 cubes at the edge of the table, places a 3rd cube within easy reach on the table, and offers the child a 4th. She may point to the 3rd cube, and she may dismantle and replace the demonstration tower once or twice to induce performance. Finally, the infant may be permitted to remove the tower cube, but initially the demonstration tower should be out of reach.

11. Massed Cubes

12–56 Weeks Maturity. The examiner arranges the 10 cubes into a square of 9 with the 10th cube surmounting the mass, and the cubes are advanced into position. Cubes that the infant pushes to the platform or floor are retrieved later; cubes that are pushed out of reach on the table may be moved nearer. If necessary, the infant may be helped to grasp a cube.

48–56 Weeks Maturity. If the tower building was not elicited during the Tower of Two situation (above), another attempt may be made to elicit this behavior.

15–36 Months Maturity. The cubes are placed in position, and the child is asked to "make something." His spontaneous exploitation of the cubes is observed.

12. Tower

15–36 Months Maturity. While the child is holding a cube, the examiner points to a cube on the table, saying, *"Put it here."* If the child does not comply, the examiner may start the tower by placing 1 or more cubes. Each time the child places a cube successfully, or at appropriate intervals, he is praised, *"Good!,"* and encouraged to continue. If the child has difficulty with precise release but clearly understands the concept of building, the examiner may hold each succeeding cube the *child* himself puts into position.

13. Train

18–30 Months Maturity. The examiner says, *"I'll show you how to make a choo-choo train,"* and removes all the cubes. He then shows the child how to align 4 cubes, saying, *"This is one car, another car and another car."* He pushes his train across the table, saying, *"Choo-choo-choo,"* then dismantles the model and shoves the disarranged cubes toward the child, saying, *"You make it."*

14. Train with Chimney.

24–36 Months Maturity. The examiner says, *"Now I'll show you a fancy choo-choo train,"* and removes all the cubes. As in the Train situation, she comments as she shows the child how to align 4 cubes and then places a 5th on top of an end cube, saying, *"These are the cars; this is the chimney for smoke to come out."* She again pushes her train across the table, saying, *"Choo-choo-choo,"* dismantles the model and shoves the disarranged cubes toward the child, saying, *"You make it."* If the child fails to place the chimney, she may ask, *"Where is the chimney?"*

COPYING from a model is more advanced behavior which the child should be given the opportunity to do first. IMITATION of a task which the examiner has demonstrated is less advanced and should be given after copying.

15. Bridge ■■■

36 + Months Maturity: Copying. Behind a screen, or opportunistically while the child is still occupied with the train, the examiner builds a 3-cube bridge and says, *"See the house I've made. It has a downstairs, an upstairs and a door,"* pointing to each of the blocks and the separation in turn. Leaving the model in place, he gives the child 3 cubes, saying, *"You make it down here."*

30–36 Months Maturity: Imitation. The examiner says, *"Now I'll show you how to make a little house." "One like this, one like this and one like this,"* as she places each block in turn. *"See, it has a downstairs, an upstairs and a door,"* again pointing to each block in turn. She leaves the model in place and gives the child 3 cubes, saying, *"You make it down here."*

16. Cup

12–16 Weeks Maturity. The cubes are removed and the cup is presented upright with the handle pointing directly toward the child. This situation is omitted if the infant already has contacted any of the cubes.

17. Cup and Cubes

24-48 Weeks Maturity. When the infant picks up at least 1 of the massed cubes, attention is called to the upright cup tapped at the edge of the tabletop. The cup then is placed within reach alongside the massed cubes, and the spontaneous play is observed. After *28 weeks,* when the infant has a cube in hand, the examiner points into the cup, saying, *"Put it in there."* If there is no compliance, the examiner takes a cube and, after securing the infant's attention, drops the cube into the cup. Responses are then observed.

48 Weeks–24 Months Maturity. The cup is added within reach alongside the mass of cubes. If the child does not begin to insert the cubes, the examiner says, *"Put the blocks in."* If the child hesitates, or starts removing the cubes after a few are inserted, he says, *"More,"* *"Put them all in,"* and pushes 1 cube after another toward the child by way of proffer. The examiner may pick up and hold cubes out to the child, or gently inhibit their removal from the cup. When all cubes have been put into the cup, he holds out his hands and says, *"Give me the cup."*

18. Cube and Paper

40–48 Weeks Maturity. A cube is tapped at the edge of the table to secure the infant's attention. While the infant looks at the cube, the examiner covers it with a piece of onionskin paper. He lifts the paper off the cube and calls attention to it once or twice. The cube covered with the paper then is pushed within the infant's reach, with *"Find the block," "Go get the toy," "Where is it?"*

48–56 Weeks Maturity. While the infant watches, the examiner places a cube in the center of a piece of onionskin paper, brings the 4 corners of the paper together and gently twists the paper to cover the cube and make a small bundle. It is given to the infant. A request is made to *"Find the block."* If the infant does not respond, the examiner unwraps the cube while the infant watches, rewraps it, and hands it back to the infant.

19. Cup and Cube

44–52 Weeks Maturity. A cube is tapped at the edge of the table to secure the infant's attention. While the infant looks at the cube, the examiner covers it with a cup, with the handle pointing toward the infant. He lifts the cup off the cube and calls attention to it once or twice. The cube covered with the cup then is pushed within the infant's reach, with *"Find the block," "Go get the toy," "Where is it?"*

20. Pellet

12–52 Weeks Maturity. The examiner presents the pellet, flat side up. If it is hit from position, it is restored. The examiner intervenes, if possible, before the infant carries the pellet to her mouth. If the infant is too quick, the mother is reassured that the pellet is edible. Sooner or later, infants usually let the pellet slip out of the mouth, when it can be removed. The examiner may attempt to call the infant's attention to the pellet by tapping her finger near it. She must withdraw her hand slowly, since the younger infants tend to follow the moving hand. Usually it is best to wait until the infant spies the pellet spontaneously.

21. Pellet Beside Bottle

32–48 Weeks Maturity. The examiner places the pellet and the bottle on the tabletop 2 to 3 inches apart, the pellet at the infant's right. He calls attention to the pellet, then to the bottle and to the pellet again, tapping back and forth. Pushing the pellet with thumb and index finger of his left hand and the bottle with his right hand, the examiner brings both simultaneously within reach and observes the spontaneous behavior. If the infant picks up only the bottle, attention may be directed toward the pellet again while the infant holds the bottle. As in the Pellet situation, the examiner should forestall the infant from eating the pellet. At *48 weeks* the examiner asks the child to put the pellet in the bottle, demonstrating if necessary.

52 Weeks-21 Months Maturity. The examiner presents the pellet and bottle simultaneously, placing them side by side on the tabletop within the child's reach, the pellet at the child's right. The child is asked to put the pellet in the bottle; demonstration may be needed. After he or the child has inserted the pellet, the examiner says, "*Get it out,*" "*Get the candy,*" demonstrating dumping if necessary. If the examiner is trying to induce placing the pellet into the bottle, the pellet is left beside the bottle following any demonstration; conversely, if he is trying to elicit dumping the pellet out, it is left inside the bottle.

22. Pellet in Bottle

32–44 Weeks Maturity. The examiner takes the top of the bottle in her left hand and holds it so the bottom is at about the level of the infant's eyes. The pellet, in the right hand, is held over the mouth of the bottle. After securing the infant's attention to the pellet in hand, she drops it into the bottle. The bottle then is placed on the table with the pellet visible to the infant, or she is allowed to take it from the examiner. If the pellet does not fall out of the bottle during exploitation, the examiner simulates this by tossing one on the tabletop, making sure that the infant does not see her do it.

23. 10 Pellets and Bottle

30–36+ Months Maturity. 10 pellets and the bottle are placed before the child, the pellets to the side of the preferred hand. "*Put them all in the bottle just as fast as you can, but one at a time.*" Repeat instructions if the child dawdles or grasps several pellets at once. The time taken to complete the task is recorded, *provided* the pellets are put in singly. The pellets then are placed on the other side of the bottle and use of the dominant hand is inhibited, unless this results in vigorous protest or refusal.

24. Bell

16–44 Weeks Maturity. The bell is presented, without being rung, and placed upright on the tabletop. At *16 and 20 weeks* the infant may need help to grasp it, and it always may be restored if dropped. Ringing is demonstrated if necessary; this requires a broad sweep of the examiner's whole arm.

25. Ring-String

24–56 Weeks Maturity. The examiner, holding the ring in the left hand with the end of the string in the right, pulls the string taut. The ring is placed out of reach at the far edge of the table, the end of the string within reach obliquely toward the infant's right. The string is held in place on the table and attention called to the ring by tapping it up and down. If the string is flipped out of position it may be restored. If the string is ignored in the oblique position, it may be placed with the end of the string directly in front of the infant. If he is unable to secure the ring and threatens to cry, it is moved within reach. At *48–56 weeks*, dangling of the ring may be demonstrated, using an up-and-down movement and broad sweeps of the arm.

26. Yarn

12–20 Weeks Maturity. The infant's attention is called to the yarn which is held suspended above the tabletop in the line of vision in the midline. Once attention is secured, the examiner moves the suspended ball slowly from one side to the other, in an arc of 180°.

12–24 Weeks Maturity. The examiner calls the infant's attention to the ball of yarn placed at the infant's right-hand edge of the tabletop. The yarn is pulled slowly across the table and finally allowed to drop off the edge toward the floor.

27. Pegboard

44 Weeks–24 Months Maturity. The pegboard is placed in front of the child and the examiner begins with the large round peg, followed by the small round, large square, and small square. He inserts and replaces the peg once or twice. The peg is left in the hole and the child is urged to take it out. At *56 weeks–24 months* the child also is urged to put it back in. The same procedure is repeated with the rest of the pegs.

28. Toy and Stick

56 Weeks–24 Months Maturity. The toy and stick are presented so that the child cannot reach the toy with her hand. She can reach it by using the stick. The stick is handed to the child if necessary and she is restrained from climbing on the table to get the "dog." The examiner requests, *"Go get the doggie," "Make the doggie come to you."* If the child does not respond, the examiner encourages, *"Use the stick."* The examiner then may demonstrate, pulling the toy toward the child with the stick, saying, *"Here comes the doggie,"* repeating the movement once or twice. The toy and stick then are placed in their original positions.

29. Safety Pin and Shoelace

24–30 Months Maturity. The examiner holds the safety pin in 1 hand and the end of the shoelace in the other. As he inserts the end of the shoelace through the hole in the safety pin, he says, *"See what I am doing?" "It goes through here just like this."* The maneuver is repeated once or twice. The examiner then places the safety pin in a favorable position in 1 of the child's hands, and places the end of the shoelace in the fingertips of the child's other hand. He encourages, *"Put it in."*

30. Beads

30–36 Months Maturity. The tube filled with the beads is shown to the child and the beads are dumped onto the table. The child is told, *"Put them back."* If the child does not succeed spontaneously, the examiner holds the tube in 1 hand and slowly lowers the dangled beads into it. She then dumps the beads on the table again and tells the child to put them back.

31. Scissors

30–36 Months Maturity. Using the same paper as for the Drawing situations, the examiner makes 1 or 2 cuts in a piece of paper, saying, *"You do it just like this."* He then sets the scissors down next to the paper and encourages the child to cut.

MIRROR SITUATIONS

32. Mirror

12–56 Weeks Maturity. The roller shade is lifted, and the infant is turned around to face the mirror. If the supporting chair has been used, the infant is removed and firm support around her chest is maintained by the examiner. She should sit or be held very close to the mirror. If the infant stares at her feet or the image of her feet, the examiner may tap the glass to call attention to the infant's face.

33. Mirror and Ball

48–56 Weeks Maturity. While the infant is looking in the mirror, the small ball is held behind him so that its image is visible in the mirror, and his reaction is noted. If there is no response to the image of the ball, bring it slowly forward until he turns his head to look at it, as a gross test for visual fields. He then is given the ball to hold in his hand and exploit. If the infant has difficulty retaining the ball, substitute the ring.

DRAWING SITUATIONS

In these situations, if the child objects to releasing the crayon, the examiner may use a second crayon. After each demonstration, he must conceal this crayon. Each demonstration should have the child's attention and be made so the child can see what is being done. Each demonstration should be done on a fresh side or piece of paper.

34. Spontaneous Drawing

15–36 Months Maturity. A piece of paper at least 5 by 8 inches is placed on the table directly before the child. The examiner steadies the paper, unless the child objects, and places the crayon in the center of the paper, pointing away from the child. The child is asked to "*Write on the paper,*" or to "*Make something.*" At *24–36 months* she is asked to *name* what she has made. The crayon is handed to the child if she does not pick it up.

35. Scribble Imitation

48 Weeks–18 Months Maturity. The examiner takes the crayon from the child and turns over the paper if the child has been marking it. After securing the child's attention, and holding his arm elevated so that his arm and hand do not obstruct the child's view, the examiner marks back and forth several times across the top of the paper with well-defined strokes. He then replaces the crayon in a central position, saying, "*You make it.*" He may put it in the child's hand in such a position that, when the child pronates, the point of the crayon contacts the paper.

36. Vertical Stroke

30–36+ Months Maturity: Copying. The examiner shows the child a card on which a vertical stroke has been drawn, saying, *"Make one like this"* (pointing) *"on your paper"* (pointing). If the child's response is unsatisfactory, the vertical stroke is demonstrated.

52 Weeks–24 Months Maturity: Imitation. The examiner takes the child's crayon, draws a decisive stroke down the left margin of the paper, and releases the crayon centrally, saying, *"You do it. Make one just like this."* The stroke movement may be slightly exaggerated. Rapid and slow movements may be tried and more than one stroke made to induce imitation.

37. Circular Scribble Imitation

18–24 Months Maturity. The examiner takes the child's crayon and makes a decisive circular scribble, going round and round at the top of the page. He releases the crayon, saying, *"You make it."* (Note: the words "circles" and "round" are never used unless the child says them first.)

38. Horizontal Stroke

30–36+ Months Maturity: Copying. The examiner shows the child a card on which a horizontal stroke has been drawn, saying, *"Make one like this"* (pointing) *"on your paper"* (pointing). If the child's response is unsatisfactory, the horizontal stroke is demonstrated.

24–36 Months Maturity: Imitation. The examiner takes the child's crayon and draws a decisive stroke acrosss the top margin of the paper, releases the crayon and says, *"You make it. Make it just like this."* Rapid and slow strokes and more than one are tried, as for the vertical stroke. When they are included, the Horizontal Stroke situations follow the respective Vertical Stroke situations (36).

39. Circle

30–36+ Months Maturity: Copying. The examiner shows the child a card on which a circle has been drawing, saying, *"Make one like this"* (pointing) *"on your paper"* (pointing). If the child's response is unsatisfactory, the circle is demonstrated, followed by the Circular Scribble situation (37).

24–36 Months Maturity: Imitation. The examiner takes the child's crayon and makes a single circle on a piece of paper. He releases the crayon, saying, *"You make it."* (Note: the words "circle" and "round" are never used unless the child says them first.)

40. Cross

30–36 Months Maturity: Imitation. The examiner takes the child's crayon and makes a decisive cross at the top of the paper, vertical stroke first, saying with each stroke, *"One like this, and one like that."* She releases the crayon, saying, *"You make it."* (Note: The cross is never named unless the child says it first.)

41. Incomplete Man

30–36 Months Maturity. The sheet with the outline of the Incomplete Man is placed before the child and he is asked, *"What is this?"* *"What do you call it?"* At this age he is unlikely to add any parts, even if they are indicated to him.

FORM PERCEPTION SITUATIONS

42. Formboard

The examiner always places the formboard on the table before the child with the round hole at the child's right, the apex of the triangular hole centered to the child's body and pointing away from the child.

44–52 Weeks Maturity. The examiner holds the formboard securely on the table with her left hand and with her right offers the infant the round block, presenting it centrally. After the infant has looked over the board and manipulated the block, the examiner points to the round hole, saying, *"Put it in."* If there is no response the examiner takes the round block and ostentatiously inserts it into the hole. If the infant cannot remove it, the examiner demonstrates how to lift one edge up with her thumb. Finally, the examiner takes the block out, restores it to the infant and again tries to induce insertion or removal.

56 Weeks–15 Months Maturity. The examiner holds the formboard securely on the table with her left hand and with her right offers the child the round block, presenting it centrally. After the child has manipulated the block, the examiner points to the round hole, saying, *"Put it in."* Either the child or finally the examiner inserts the block. The examiner then says, *"Watch what I'm doing,"* lifts the board, leaving the block on the table, and turns the board slowly through an arc of 180°, keeping it flat. As she releases the board on the table, she shoves the block to the table edge at the right. The round block is now on the table directly in front of the square hole. If the child does not pick up the block, the examiner offers it centrally, saying, *"Put it in."* The examiner may point to the correct hole if the child fails to respond, or place the block herself before repeating the rotation.

15 Months Maturity. The examiner holds the formboard securely on the table with her left hand and with his right offers the child the square block, presenting it centrally. After the child has manipulated the block, the examiner points to the square hole, saying, *"Put it in."* If the child does not respond appropriately, the examiner demonstrates the insertion of the square block, removes it and hands it back to the child, again making a request to *"Put it in."* The examiner may help in adjusting the corners.

18–36 Months Maturity. The examiner places the formboard on the table and puts the 3 blocks in front of their respective holes between the board and the child. *"Put the blocks in."* Before the examiner makes any further moves, the child's spontaneous behavior with each of the 3 blocks in turn is observed. If the child has difficulty in adjusting corners in insertion, she may be assisted. If she piles all 3 blocks, then insertion is demonstrated, the examiner patting each block into place, and the situation is presented again. The examiner may point to the proper holes to induce placement. When all 3 blocks are in, the examiner lifts the board, leaving the 3 blocks on the table, and turns the board slowly through an arc of 180°, saying, *"Watch!"* In this maneuver she keeps the board flat. As she replaces the board on the table, she shoves the blocks back toward the edge of the table. The round block is now on the table directly in front of the square hole and vice versa. *"Put them in again—nicely."* If the child makes an error and persists in it, the examiner may say, *"Where does it go?"* The examiner then may run her fingers back and forth on the far side of the board and fianlly point to the correct hole. Three or 4 trials may be given.

43. Vertical Slot or Performance Box

18–24 Months Maturity. The examiner sets the vertical slot form or the performance box on the table in front of the child and hands him the square block. If the child does not bring it to the hole, the examiner encourages, *"Put it in,"* *"All the way,"* *"Turn it around so it fits."* If necessary, the examiner completes or starts the insertion. The child again is handed the block in a manner so that he must make a manual adjustment to insert it. He is told, *"Do it again."* If failure threatens to annoy the child, help him insert it. If the child holds the square block in his own right hand, the face of the form is angled toward his right hand; conversely, if he uses his left hand, insertion is facilitated by angling the form toward his left hand. It may be necessary to shift the form from one position to the other as the child transfers the block.

44. Color Forms

24–36 Months Maturity. The color card is placed on the table, the circle in the upper right corner, and the child's attention is called to the forms on the card with, *"Look at all my pictures."* She is given the cut-out round form and asked, *"Where does it go?,"* *"You put it on."* If she misplaces it or fails to place it, the examiner demonstrates and allows the child to place it. She then is given, in order, the square, triangle, semicircle, and cross. Vary the instructions: *"Look at all of them on the paper,"* *"Put it where it fits,"* *"Put it right on top of the one that looks just like it."* The round form is the only one demonstrated; all other placements or pointings are accepted by the examiner, who merely says, *"Good,"* after each response, whether right or wrong.

45. Geometric Forms

36+ Months Maturity. The card with the 10 geometric forms is placed before the child and the matching circle is laid on the X in the bottom row or handed to the child. *"Where is the other one?"* *"Show me the other one just like this."* *"Where does this one go?"* If the child fails to indicate or incorrectly indicates the circle, the examiner points to it. The child may be allowed to place the test form on its corresponding one on the card. The circle is the only one demonstrated; all other placements or pointings are accepted by the examiner, who merely says, *"Good,"* after each response, whether right or wrong. Present in order the circle, square, triangle, oval, rectangle, hexagon, rhomboid, square with indented arc, trapezoid and irregular.

VERBAL SITUATIONS

If the child fails to talk, the examiner should omit all the verbal situations except those requiring only pointing or action responses.

Always ask the child to make the verbal response first. If it is clear that the child cannot or will not respond, the situations are not prolonged.

46. Picture Book

52 Weeks–36 Months Maturity. At *56 weeks,* the examination begins at this point. The picture book *Goosey Gander* is put on the table, and the examiner starts by describing what is on the cover. She then may call attention to the salient features on each page, may ask for comments and responses on each page, or may skip through the book rapidly. The situation is used to introduce the examination, to get the child talking, if she will, or to give the examiner a chance to disarm the child by responding for her. The examiner may ask the child to turn pages or to complete the turn she starts; the examiner may need to do all the turning.

At *52 WEEKS–24 MONTHS* the child is asked first to *name* and then to *point* to shoes, hat, dog, spoon, baby, umbrella, etc. If the child fails to name or point, the examiner herself points.

At *24–36 MONTHS* the child is asked to *tell* and then to *indicate* what the child is doing (crying, eating, sleeping). Again the examiner answers her own questions if need be.

At *36 MONTHS* she may be asked to recite a familiar nursery rhyme, with or without help.

47. Body Parts

15–30 Months Maturity. The examiner shows the child the doll, and while pointing to the doll's eyes, asks, "*What's this? . . . Dolly's what?*" If the child does not respond, the examiner repeats the question for one or two more body parts. If there still is no response, the examiner asks the child to *identify* body parts, saying, "*Show me the dolly's eyes,*" "*Put your finger on the dolly's eyes,*" (nose, mouth, hands, feet, hair, ears). If the child does not respond on the doll, the examiner makes the same request for him to point on his own, his mother's or the examiner's body. Any 7 body parts acceptable.

48. Picture Cards

18–36 Months Maturity. The card with 4 pictures is presented, the examiner retaining the card. The examiner points to each picture, asking, "*What is this?,*" in the following order: (1) dog, (2) shoe, (3) cup, (4) house. For any the child does not name, ask in the same order, "*Where is the doggie (or bow-wow)?,*" "*Show me where it is.*"

If the child fails to name or point, the examiner may point before proceeding to the next situation.

24–36 Months Maturity. The examiner says, *"Here are some more pictures,"* presenting the card with 6 pictures and retaining it. The examiner points to the pictures, asking, *"What is this?,"* in the following order: (1) clock, (2) basket, (3) book, (4) flag, (5) leaf, (6) star. For any the child does not name, ask in the same order, *"Where is the clock (tick-tock)?"* If she does not respond to the first 2 or 3 pictures, the remainder are omitted.

49. Name and Sex

36 + Months Maturity. The examiner says, *"What is your name?"* If the child does not respond or gives only his first name (or nickname), the examiner says, *"(Johnny) what?"* A response never is insisted upon. The examiner then says to a girl, *"Are you a (little) girl or a (little) boy?;"* to a boy, *"Are you a (little) boy or a (little) girl?"* He may also say, *"Which are you?,"* if the response is unsatisfactory. Do not say, *"Are you a girl?"* If the question is to be repeated, give the full form.

50. Comprehension Questions A

36 + Months Maturity. The examiner asks, in order: *"What do you do when you are hungry?" "What do you do when you are sleepy?" "What do you do when you are cold?"*

51. Digits

30–36 + Months Maturity. If the child is giving verbal responses fairly freely, say to him, *"Listen, say 4–2," "Good," "Now say 6–3."* The numbers should be recited in a spaced manner. The following digit series are used: 4–7, 6–3, 5–8, 6–4–1, 3–5–2, 8–3–7, 4–7–2–9, 3–8–5–2, 7–2–6–1. Do not repeat a series. If necessary, ask the child to wait until you have finished, with, *"I am going to say all the numbers first and when I am through I want you to say them." "Listen carefully."*

52. Test Objects

18–24 Months Maturity: Names. The examiner shows the child the following objects in order: pencil, shoe (the examiner's), key and penny, saying, *"What is this?"* If there is no response, place the pencil, key and penny on the table in front of the child, and ask for 1 of the objects. Whether the response is correct or not, replace the objects she has given to you and juggle the position of the objects on the table. Continue to ask for different test objects, juggling their position each time to avoid hand or position preference. The examiner retains possession of all the objects. If the *18–21 month* child does not respond to the first 2 objects, skip to the Small Ball situations after asking her to name the ball.

30–36 Months Maturity: Use. If the child names or identifies an object correctly, say, "*What do you do with it?*" The child who does not talk may pantomine a correct response.

53. Action Agents

36+ Months Maturity. The examiner begins by asking, "*What runs?*" If the child does not respond, the examiner continues with, "*Does a doggie run?*," "*Does a car run?*" He gives a second example if necessary, "*What cries?*," "*Does a baby cry?*" He continues, asking the following agents: "*What flies, bites, sleeps, scratches, swims, cuts, burns, blows, shoots, boils, sails, melts, floats, growls, gallops, stings, aches, explodes, roars, meows?*," stopping when it is obvious the child is not responding correctly.

54. Colors

36+ Months Maturity. Place 4 small blocks, wooden beads or other identical objects of red, blue, green, and yellow on the table. Pointing to each in turn, ask, "*What color is this?*"

If there is no correct response say to the child, "*Give me the red one.*" Whatever her response, replace the object on the table and ask for the next one. If in doubt about the response, repeat until you are sure whether or not the child identifies any of the colors.

CONCEPTS

55. Big and Little

30–36 Months Maturity. The examiner puts the big and little blocks on the table, saying, "*See these blocks. They are the same color but one is big and one is little.*" He requests, "*Give me the BIG block,*" saying, "*Thank you,*" regardless of the child's response. If the child responds correctly, the examiner then points to the little one and asks, *"What is this one?"* If the child answers correctly, the situation is finished. If he does not answer, the blocks are juggled and the examiner asks for the little block or the big one until the child's responses are clear.

56. Up and Down

30–36 Months Maturity. The examiner presents the open-faced box with a bead on a string. Beginning with the bead in a central position, she moves it up and down, saying, *"See, I can move this bead up and down."* She leaves the bead in a central position and cautions the child, *"I'm going to tell you which way to move it," "Move it jut UP."* The examiner moves the bead back to a central position after the child has responded. She varies the "up" and "down" requests to insure that the child is not responding to the last placed position of the bead, and she continues until the child's responses are clear.

57. Loud and Soft

36+ Months Maturity. The examiner, presenting the loud and soft containers, shakes first one and then the other while saying, *"I have a LOUD one and a SOFT one."* The examiner then juggles the containers and hands one to each of the child's hands. He tells the child to shake first one and then other, then requests, *"Give me the LOUD one."* If the child hands the correct container, the examiner points to the soft one and asks, *"What is that one?"* If the child answers correctly, the situation is finished. If he does not answer, the containers are juggled and handed back to the child and the examiner asks for the loud or the soft until the child's responses are clear.

SMALL BALL

58. Ball Play

48 Weeks–15 Months Maturity. The test table is removed; the child remains seated on the crib or on her mother's lap at the adjustable table. The examiner retreats a short distance and casts the ball to the child, helping her to grasp it if necessary. The examiner then holds out her hands and asks the child to throw the ball. She may take it and bounce it away from the child and back again once or twice to induce responsive release.

15–36 Months Maturity. The child has just been given an opportunity to name the ball. She is given the ball and the table is moved aside so that she is free to get up and walk around. The examiner holds out her hand and says, *"Throw it."* It sometimes helps if the examiner squats down to the child's level.

59. Directions with Ball

15–24 Months Maturity. The examiner squats down, secures the child's attention, and gives him the ball, saying, *"Now we are going to play a game with the ball," "Don't throw it," "Put the ball on the TABLE."* The request may be repeated several times, but an incorrect response is accepted with, *"Good."* Secure the ball again, and give it to the child, saying, *"Put it on the CHAIR."* Then, warning the mother not to hold out her hands, *"Give it to MOTHER."* Then, *"Give it to ME," "Thank you."* If necessary, add, *"I'll give it back to you."* If he insists on throwing the ball, substitute a block or similar object.

60. Ball in Basket or Box

18–21 Months Maturity. The examiner holds the performance box or wastebasket upright on the floor, tips the open end toward the child, and invites her to throw the ball in. *"Get it out."* Safeguard the child when she leans into the box, when she lifts it and sets it down, and when she pulls it over. She may be recalled to the task if she abandons it. If she is unsuccessful, the examiner says, *"Turn the box over."* She may demonstrate and finally get the ball for the child. (Note: A very tall child can reach the ball, invalidating the situation. It may be given to a short 24-month old.)

61. Prepositions with Ball

30–36 Months Maturity. The child has just thrown the ball. The examiner takes the ball and gives it to the child, saying, *"We are going to play a game," "Put the ball ON the chair,"* then, *"Put it UNDER the chair."* An incorrect response is accepted and the *Directions with Ball situation* (59) given. Follow correct responses with additional prepositions: in back of (behind), in front of, beside.

POSTURAL SITUATIONS

After *56 weeks*, the postural tests are so free as to be incidental rather than imposed formally. During the interview the child may have demonstrated most of his gross motor capacities. Items 69, 72, and 73 are exceptions to this rule. If the infant of *36–56 weeks* is in the crib or on the floor during the interview, he also may demonstrate most of his locomotor abilities, and they need not be elicited formally. From

4 to 52 weeks, the infant's shoes and stockings are removed prior to the examination and the remainder of his clothes are not taken off until the postural situations, unless they interfere with his manipulation. From *56 weeks to 36 months,* he keeps his clothes throughout all situations. Depending on the indications, they then may be removed for further observation of locomotion and any necessary physical examination.

62. Sitting Supported

Note: This should be carried out on a *hard* surface.

4–20 Weeks Maturity. After the infant has been pulled to sitting or turned away from the mirror, the examiner squats down to the infant's eye level and supports her by the sides of the thorax. Sitting posture and control are observed; the examiner may release her support slightly to determine the infant's participation in the sitting act. Of course, the infant should neither be permitted to fall nor to lean too far forward, nor should this be at all prolonged.

24–32 Weeks Maturity. At the conclusion of the mirror situation, the examiner turns the infant on the platform, squats down to the infant's eye level, and removes her hands from the infant's chest, though they remain protectively near. If necessary, the infant's legs should be arranged in a diamond shape and her hands placed in a propping position alongside her feet. If she maintains her balance, a lure may be offered to test her ability to lift one hand and still maintain position, and to induce, if possible, an erect sitting position. The examiner is on the alert to protect the infant from losing her balance.

63. Standing Supported

4–20 Weeks Maturity. The infant has been sitting, supported by a hand on either side of the chest. The examiner now lifts the infant to the standing position, holding him securely under the arms. He releases his support slightly to ascertain the infant's participation in the standing act. At *28 weeks,* the examiner shifts his hands, one at a time, and holds the infant's hands at shoulder height with elbows fully extended to provide only balance, not support.

64. Ventral Suspension

4–20 Weeks Maturity. The examiner has been holding the standing infant facing her. She now turns the infant away from her and adjusts her hands from behind so that her right hand is under the infant's right arm, the left under the left. She suspends the infant horizontally face down over the crib and observes her postural compensation as she is lowered to the platform.

65. Prone

4–20 Weeks Maturity. After he is placed on the platform following ventral suspension, adjust the infant's arms if necessary so they are not caught under his chest or extended footward. If the infant does not turn and lift his head, the examiner takes the head between his hands and gently turns it so that the infant's chin rests on the table. If the head lifts, dangle a lure before his eyes, raising it to induce optimal head lifting. Do not prolong this situation if there is any protest. At this age range, this situation concludes the examination.

24–28 Weeks Maturity. The infant has rolled to or is placed in the prone position on the crib platform by the maneuver described above. Dangle a lure before his eyes, raising it to induce optimal head lifting. Then put the lure on the platform just out of reach at the side; as the infant *pivots*, keep the lure just out of reach. Try one side then the other. When the infant has exhibited his abilities while prone, reward him with the lure.

28–52 Weeks Maturity. The infant either is placed prone or has attained the prone position himself. Using a lure kept just out of reach, try to induce *creeping* forward. At *24–28 weeks* this situation concludes the examination.

66. Sitting Free

32–52 Weeks Maturity. The infant sits on the crib platform or other *hard* surface. After her sitting posture has been observed, place the lure on the platform before her, just out of reach. Observe her ability to either lean forward and reerect herself or go over to the prone position.

52 Weeks–36 Months Maturity. The child's ability to seat herself in an ordinary *small* kindergarten *chair* and to get up again are noted, either at the beginning of the examination or opportunistically.

67. Railing

32–48 Weeks Maturity. If he does not creep over to the crib rail, the infant is placed seated, facing it. The examiner dangles a lure at the top of the rail, just out of reach, to induce the standing position. If necessary, place the infant's hands on the rail; the mother may dangle the lure and call him. If he does not pull to his feet at the rail, place him standing so that he may hold the rail, and then release support. At *32 and 36 weeks*, this situation concludes the examination.

36–48 Weeks Maturity. While the infant is standing holding the crib rail, dangle the lure just out of reach to the side. If the infant steps sideward, keep the lure out of reach. Try one side, then the other. When her cruising ability has been observed, place the lure down on the platform of the crib and observe the infant's efforts to secure the toy while holding the railing, and also to lower herself to sitting again.

68. Walking Supported

44–52 Weeks Maturity. The examiner takes the infant's hands and tries to induce him to walk. Many infants will perform better if allowed on the floor at this time; some will do better if the mother holds the hands. If he walks when both hands are supported at shoulder height, or overhead just for balance, try releasing one hand. At *40–48 weeks*, this situation concludes the examination.

69. Large Ball

18–36 Months Maturity. After the small ball is removed, the large ball is handed to the child. After she has thrown it once or twice, it is placed on the floor before her and she is asked to *"Kick it," "Give it a good kick," "Kick it with your foot."* The examiner may take the hand of a younger child if she does not respond, and repeat the request. If she responds with the hand held, release her hand and repeat the request again. The examiner also may demonstrate kicking if the child does not respond; she must use a wide swing of the leg. (Note: The child should be in the center of the room so that she cannot hold wall or furniture to steady herself.)

70. Walking, Running

52 Weeks Maturity. Seat the child on the floor and use a lure to induce him to stand up and take steps to secure it. The mother may be successful in eliciting the response.

56 Weeks–36 Months Maturity. Running and walking are observed incidentally during the interview or ball situations.

71. Stairs

52 Weeks–36+ Months Maturity. If stairs are available and the behavior has not been observed opportunistically prior to the examination, encourage the child to creep up and down, or to walk up and down in the erect position, holding her hand when it is indicated. At *52 weeks–21 months,* this situation concludes the examination.

72. Standing

24–36+ Months Maturity. Lead the child to the center of the room so that he cannot hold wall or furniture for support. Stand facing the child and say, *"Stand on one foot like this," "Pick up your foot."* The examiner demonstrates and encourages, *"That's the way!," "Keep it up."* Showing the child how to hold dress or pants with both hands facilitates the performance. When the child lifts his foot, the examiner may time the performance in an approximate way by counting *"1–2–3"* at the rate of 1 per second.

73. Jumping

24–36 Months Maturity. The examiner jumps in place with both feet off the floor, saying, *"You do what I'm doing."* If stairs are available, ask the child to jump off the bottom step. Occasionally an equivalent height is available for this purpose. At *36 months* the examiner demonstrates a broad jump using both feet at once, saying, *"You do what I'm doing."* This concludes the examination.

5
Differential Diagnosis

Normal development is dependent upon an intact organism; disease, defects, or damage that impair the integrity of the organism deflect the normal currents of development. A knowledge of normal development is the basis on which the detection and elucidation of abnormality rests, and it is essential to the diagnosis of intellectual, motor, sensory and other deviations. The objective of differential developmental diagnosis is the prevention, cure, or amelioration of the adverse consequences of developmental deviations.

The ensuing brief summaries of developmental abnormalities and of the variety of clinical entities will illustrate that quantification of behavior is but one aspect of diagnosis. They have been drawn from the fuller discussions in Chapters 5–16 of Developmental Diagnosis; *reference should be made to those chapters. When an infant or young child with abnormal signs and symptoms achieves age-appropriate behavior, more weight must be given to the abnormalities in arriving at a diagnosis. Each facet of behavior makes its own unique contribution to the evaluation of neuropsychologic function. For adequate diagnosis and prognosis, the distinctions must be appreciated to do justice to the complexity and variability of early development.*

INTELLECTUAL POTENTIAL

An understanding of mental subnormality is fundamental to differential clinical diagnosis. In all cases of defective and deviant development, the first inquiry is whether the consequent retardations and deformations of behavior are deep-seated or transient, generalized or delimited, ameliorable or irreducible. Mental deficiency must be recognized and ruled out.

150

Mental subnormality is defined as subnormal general intellectual functioning which originates during the developmental period and is associated with impairment of either learning and social adjustment, or maturation, or both. It is extremely important to recognize that subnormal intelligence is composed of two distinct categories, which may overlap. In one instance, the subnormality is a result of some pathologic condition of the brain which precludes normal development, and properly is referred to as *mental deficiency*. *Mental retardation* is a term which should be reserved for indivduals who function below their potential level of ability; it is usually the result of suboptimum environmental situations, and not due to organic central nervous system disease. Today the term mental retardation has replaced all previously applied terms and is the one used and understood by professionals and the laity alike. The following discussion, however, maintains the distinction.

MENTAL DEFICIENCY

Mental deficiency *is evidence* of organic disease of the brain, and impairs that aspect of function most uniquely human. It is manifested by an impairment of developmental potentials. As a consequence, the rate of maturation is retarded, and the ultimate maturity level of behavior is lowered.

If the individual's original nervous system is impaired, if it becomes damaged *in utero* or during birth, or if it is impaired by accident or disease after birth, he cannot meet adequately the demands of his environment, even in infancy. Thus, a mentally deficient person is one who will *always* require some degree of special care and help for his own social welfare and for that of his family and of others. Every diagnosis of mental deficiency in a child carries the prognostic implication that when he becomes an adult he will have some limitation in managing himself and his affairs with ordinary prudence. He will always show some lack of intelligence and independence. Impairment in social functioning in itself is not synonymous with mental deficiency, but it generally is a concomitant.

IQ AND DQ

An intelligence quotient (IQ) is an arithmetic relationship between the mental age, as measured by standard intelligence tests, and the chronologic age. Subnormal intelligence has been divided on an IQ basis as follows: profound, IQ under 20; severe, IQ 20–35; moderate, IQ 36–51; mild, IQ 52–67; borderline, IQ 68–85. (In infancy and early childhood, borderline would be defined more acceptably as 68–75.) This arbitrary psychometric classification may have descriptive, administrative, statistical and communication value, but it leads to serious errors if not used with caution in clinical situations.

Arithmetically, the developmental quotient (DQ) expresses a similar relationship between the maturity age, derived from the behavioral performance, and the actual age. Neither an IQ nor a DQ automatically delivers a diagnosis; both need qualification and interpretation. There obviously is a relationship between a clinical diagnosis and a quotient, but at no age should assignment to a broad clinical category be defined rigidly by numerical quotients. A few points in a score are not the basis for deciding if a child has "just average intelligence" or higher abilities, is mildly retarded or of borderline intelligence. Quite the contrary, if a quotient is at odds with clinical impressions of the quality and integrity of behavior, the quotient is at greater risk of being wrong, particularly in infancy. In an academically oriented professional home, an older child with a measured IQ of 85, or even 95, is clearly impaired in comparison to other family members, most likely on the basis of organic brain disease. A child in a ghetto milieu probably has no significant brain pathology and would respond to an optimum environment, in its broadest sense, and an adequate educational program. In both instances the IQ of 85 has management and treatment implications, but different ones.

Developmental diagnosis does not attempt a direct measurement of intelligence as such, but aims at clinical estimates of intellectual potential based upon an analysis of maturity status. Adaptive behavior, the forerunner of later intelligent behavior, must be the primary basis for predicting intellectual potential. Its expressions in infancy are simpler than the complex manifestations at later ages, but they are only superficially simple. For his age, the infant's integration of stimuli in a meaningful fashion is a complicated process, and is the index of the intactness of his cerebral cortex. But this adaptive behavior must always be considered in relation to the other aspects of behavior. Unlike the IQ, the DQ is not limited to a single inclusive formula. It is an adaptable device which registers changes in the growing complex of behavior. The DQ must be taken with the proverbial grain of salt. But it is infinitely more useful in the problems of diagnosis than salt alone. It takes the estimate of developmental status out of the realm of subjective impressions.

It is impossible to establish sharp distinctions between the various categories of mental deficiency. One category merges into another and, theoretically, the milder grades of mental deficiency shade into the dull-normal zone. However, it is necessary to make clear-cut distinction between mental deficiency and normality. In *infancy*, any adaptive DQ below 85 probably indicates organic impairment of some type. Whenever any DQ falls decisively below the two-thirds or three-fourths ratio (DQ 65–75), there is reason to suspect serious retardation which is a clinical indication for further study. Beyond 24–30 months, mere lowering of measured intelligence does not constitute mental deficiency if the individual shows no marked social incapacity. The diagnosis of mental deficiency should be reserved for those individuals who always will need external support and supervision because of their inadequate behavioral capacity.

MENTAL RETARDATION

Growth and development are processes of anatomic and functional integrative organization which bring "heredity" and "environment" into productive union. The manner in which an organism functions today has an effect on how it will function tomorrow. In the prediction of development, surely much depends upon what happens to a child. How much development is affected by what happens is a clinical question which always demands an estimate of developmental potentials in relationship to a given environment. Sometimes the environmental factors seem so significant that a new environment must be provided to put the question to a therapeutic test.

In appraising developmental potentials no environmental influences can be ignored: cultural milieu, siblings, parents, illness, trauma, education. But these must always be considered in relation to the organizational integrity of the child's central nervous system, which ultimately determines the degree and mode of reaction to the environment. Environmental impoverishment leads to behavioral impoverishment. It produces palpable reductions of behavior. It *does not* produce mental deficiency, but it does produce syndromes which may be severe enough to make diagnosis difficult and call for therapeutic intervention.

In the lower socioeconomic strata of society there is an increased incidence of organic mental deficiency, due to the increased incidence of many interrelated antecedent etiologic factors. Disadvantaged children are not only born *into* poverty, they are conceived *of* poverty. As a group, their mothers give evidence of malnutrition throughout their own life cycle. Maternal and infant mortality rates are increased, and there is a higher incidence of complications of pregnancy, other diseases associated with pregnancy, low birth weight, premature birth, subsequent illness, malnutrition, and lack of medical care. These biologic factors contribute to a depressed performance, and all the adverse conditions have a higher incidence in minority groups.

The largest proportion of the children, who come particularly from minority groups in this country, escape any significant injury to the central nervous system. In spite of the accumulation of adverse factors, they are without organic disease of the brain. Nevertheless, they form the largest group of children who function at a subnormal level of intellectual ability as measured by IQ and school performance. This generally depressed function on school-age tests in the lowest socioeconomic strata, and the vigor of most infants seen in well-baby clinics, have led professionals to say it is not possible to detect mild mental subnormality in infancy. The majority thus affected cannot be identified for a very simple reason: Those children with so-called "physiologic" or "familial" retardation are *normal* in infancy. Those with organic disease of the brain impairing intellectual potential, regardless of the degree of impairment or of their *social status, can* be identified in infancy. In infancy, sociocultural factors affect the psychologic level of integration through the biologic level.

At later ages, sociocultural factors have a direct effect on the psychologic level of integration. There are abundant data from many studies to indicate that the incidence of subnormality and of socioeconomic disparity in function increases with age. In infancy there are no differences with variations in race or maternal education. By 3 years and beyond there is a systematic increase in performance as the mother's education increases, with whites doing better than blacks at all maternal educational levels, because equivalent educational level does not necessarily mean equivalent education.

Improvements in measured test performance and academic achievement, associated with improved environments, have been demonstrated in a variety of situations and at different ages. A word of caution is indicated, however, in the interpretation of the test data.

The tests used in evaluating "intelligence" are not free of cultural bias. They almost always are biased in favor of the white, academically-oriented middle class and make their own contribution to the differences which are found.

The data emphasize the importance of the sociocultural milieu and its effect on the interrelationship of biologic and psychologic factors affecting development. The racial and socioeconomic phenomena have their roots in the total milieu in which children grow and develop: in medical and nutritional problems; in the noisy crowded conditions of slum living; in the lack of academic orientation in the home; in the accompanying suppression of verbal communication and curiosity; in feelings of hopelessness; and in the inferior educational facilities which usually are provided for the ghetto culture. They have definite implications for the controversy which is raging anew about the relative contributions of genetic and environmental factors to intellectual performance, not only between races, but also within each racial group.

Until optimum conditions for conception and subsequent development are provided for the entire population, it is not possible to study or define the relative contributions of "heredity" and "environment" to intellectual function. Important educational, social, and political decisions must be directed toward maximizing opportunities for each individual to develop to his fullest potential. In the present state of society, few individuals achieve this ideal goal. While man's fundamental structure, and consequently his basic functioning, is genetically determined, it is chiefly the sociocultural milieu affecting biologic and psychologic variables which modifies his behavior and, in the absence of organic brain dysfunction, makes one individual function *significantly* differently from the next.

NEUROMOTOR STATUS

Maturational status and neuromotor status are intimately interrelated. A maturity appraisal is an essential part of a neurologic diagnosis for an infant or young child. However, a clinical distinction must be drawn between signs of chronologic immaturity in motor behavior and signs of neuromotor dysfunction. The spontaneous reactions to the demands of the examination situations are the most sensitive indicators of underlying neural structure and of neuronal activity.

Functional tests of behavior define the *integrity* as well as the *maturity* of the central nervous system, and enable differentiation of normal physiologic awkwardness from neuropathologic awakwardness. The normal infant, for example, is not to be regarded as awkward. He is awkward only with respect to a very new function while it is in a nascent or assimilative stage. He has an extensive array of established functions which are executed with grace and facility. Normally he is skillful in the functions which are part and parcel of his established maturity.

THE DIAGNOSIS OF NEUROMOTOR DYSFUNCTION

Motor handicaps in infancy greatly increase the difficulty of acquiring a skill; they greatly increase the length of time needed to acquire a skill; and they exaggerate the awkwardness displayed in the nascent and assimilative stages of the development of a skill. These facts make motor handicaps readily apparent in infancy; their recognition is the first step in diagnosis.

In infants and young children the signs and symptoms of nervous system disease tend to be diffuse rather than localized. It is perhaps more important to recognize the diffuseness of the damage than its limits. This diffuseness accounts for the injuries to intellect and personality that so often accompany impairment of the neuromotor system.

Neuromotor impairments, whether mild or severe, local or general, transient or permanent, express themselves by *reduction* or *disorder* of motor performance. On the other hand, simple motor *retardation* implies a performance normal in quality, and abnormal only in terms of age. A careful distinction must be made between reduction and disorder in function, and retardation in function, even when, as is usually the case, they appear in combination.

DEGREES OF NEUROMOTOR DYSFUNCTION

When there is a qualitative change in movement control, it is generally accepted that the abnormality is due to some lesion of the central nervous system, usually demonstrable on pathologic examination. Lesser degrees of neuromotor impairment are characterized by the presence of other abnormalities in neuromotor integration which accompany such qualitative changes in movement control. There is a decreasing gradient in the frequency and pervasiveness of the signs.

The minor deviations from normal neuromotor integration are demonstrable, however, when the relationship between neuromotor integrity and maturational level is understood. For any child, his adaptive maturity level is crucial, because the diagnostic interpretation of any observed neuromotor pattern depends on the stage of his development. It is not possible to list abnormal neuromotor patterns and apply this list to all ages. The neuromotor abnormalities, the ages at which they assume diagnostic significance, and a further discussion of their recording and interpretation are found in Chapter 6.

The minor disorganizations are easiest to detect in infancy, when the rapidity of developmental changes causes lesser impairments to distort normal behavior definitively. Compensation for the disabilities occurs with increasing maturity. In the late preschool and early school period, neuromotor evaluation has not yet been formulated fully in terms of developmental stages, although increasing recognition is being given by neurologists to so-called "soft" neurologic signs.

A careful differentiation must be made between those infants and children who have abnormal neurologic integration with intellectual potential within the normal range, and those who have motor retardation—by definition, gross motor development significantly below their chronologic age *because of mental deficiency*. The motor behavior is retarded, but may be qualitatively normal for the age at which they are functioning. For the vast majority, the motor retardation is accompanied by abnormal neuromotor signs. Thus, there are parallel degrees of neuromotor dysfunction when the intellectual potential is normal and when mental deficiency is present. In the latter case, the phrase "motor retardation with" precedes the appropriate category in the first four of the five diagnostic categories of neuromotor status.

No Abnormal Neuromotor Signs. Both gross and fine motor behavior are qualitatively appropriate for the chronologic or functional age. There may be occasional or fleeting abnormal patterns, but the overall picture is well-integrated. When intellectual potential is normal, there is no interference with total performance in either motor or adaptive behavior. When mental deficiency is present, motor behavior is appropriate for the maturity level at which the child is functioning.

Abnormal Neuromotor Signs of No Clinical Importance. There are some definite abnormal patterns, which preclude a clean bill of health. However, there is no interference with total performance, and the signs are insufficient to consider them significantly outside the normal range, although technically the patterns signify some aberration.

Abnormal Neuromotor Signs of Minor Degree. There is an increase in the frequency and severity of distortions in motor integration, which usually causes delay in the rate of motor development. In those instances in which the abnormalities are chiefly unilateral motor achievements may be at age. While there often are accompanying disorders of attention, personality and integration, the term *minimal cerebral dysfunction* refers specifically to the *motor* signs. Gross compensation usually occurs by 15–18 months but the abnormalities are detected by developmental assessment.

Abnormal Neuromotor Signs of Marked Degree. The abnormal patterns are more frequent and more severe than in the previous categories, but there is no significant qualitative change in movement control. Regardless of the intellectual potential, there is greater disparity between motor and adaptive maturity levels. If the findings were present in an older child, a diagnosis of "cerebral palsy" would be made, but clinical experience indicates there is almost always gross compensation by 2 years of age. However, "cerebral palsy" cannot be ruled out definitively. At school age, abnormalities are evident by developmental assessment if motor behavior is compared with that appropriate for chronologic age.

In a few instances, the abnormal signs of minor and marked degree are precursors of various degenerative diseases of the central nervous system.

Abnormal Neuromotor Signs of Severe Degree. There are *qualitative changes in movement control and tone.* The smaller proportion of such children have space-occupying lesions, relatively clearly-defined disease processes in the spinal cord, nerve roots, or muscles, or hereditary or nonhereditary degenerative diseases. The majority suffer from a static nonprogressive insult to the brain acquired in the developmental period, between 8 weeks of gestation and 8 years of age. The term "cerebral palsy" is applied to the heterogenous group of conditions resulting from such insults. This diagnosis is made independently of the intellectual potential, although it is highly associated with mental deficiency. The rate of motor development is almost always delayed, but hemiplegics who have unquestionable unilateral disabilities may have motor achievements at age. A diagnosis of "cerebral palsy" implies that a standard neurologic examination at school age will show definite abnormality, even though it may be so mild that no treatment is required. An exception to this rule exists when hypotonia is the only manifestation of disordered movement control, since gross compensation occurs spontaneously. Then a diagnosis of "cerebral palsy" often is made erroneously, when mental deficiency is the correct diagnosis, because of failure to take into account the adaptive level at which the child is functioning.

An infant may be several months old before the exact nature of the discoordination in movement control becomes clear. Before then, however, maldevelopment of function, abnormal postures, disorders of tone, and exaggerated and abnormal reflexes are apparent, and they are indicators of neuromotor pathology. Tonal changes alone, in the presence of motor behavior which is integrated and age-appropriate, suggest a search for an acute intercurrent process or a cause outside the central nervous system.

Often it is difficult to distinguish between a performance which fails for mechanical reasons and one which fails from lack of insight and maturity. Is the child with "cerebral palsy" unable to imitate a stroke due to manual incoordination or to mental deficiency? A severely hemiplegic infant can hardly be expected to transfer a toy from hand to hand. The interpretation of each performance must rest upon its own merits. Evidences of thought or insight or effort should not be overlooked; some children will not even attempt a task when it is clearly beyond their capacities. The examiner should offer as much assistance as the child will accept, encourage effort, and even reward effort deliberately by simulating success, if these measures will help in eliciting concealed abilities. On the other hand, errors probably are made as frequently in excusing failure on grounds of motor incapacity as in penalizing a child because of motor incapacity. Errors in either direction are unfair to the child. When the motor handicap is severely incapacitating, repeated observations over a period of many months may be necessary to establish the diagnosis.

A neuromotor diagnosis has prognostic implications for maintaining normal intellectual function. When infant neuromotor status is normal or when there are abnormal neuromotor signs of no clinical importance, fewer than 5% of the previously normal infants will have an IQ of less than 75 at school age. For those with abnormal signs of minor degree, the risk of failing to maintain an IQ above 75 at school age is 25%; for those with abnormal signs of marked or severe degree, there is a 45% risk. The two most important factors in the child's subsequent life experiences in the interval appear to be the occurrence of seizures and the socioeconomic status of the family.

CONVULSIVE SEIZURE DISORDERS

The third major disorder of neuropyschologic function, seizures, figures frequently in the case histories of developmental defect and deviation. A convulsive seizure must be regarded as one of the most important symptoms in childhood. It reflects a pathologic state, and in turn may interfere directly with the normal course of development. Seizures vary enormously in immediate gravity, from a single benign episode in a fleeting infection to severe status epilepticus, a medical emergency which may terminate in death since the seizures occur in such rapid succession that the child does not regain consciousness. Seizures, *per se,* do not necessarily cause mental deterioration, but when there is loss of substrates such as glucose and oxygen, and alterations in other biochemical homeostatic mechanisms, they do cause damage and may have a devastating effect. Their recongition is vitally important because they are one of the few conditions in which proper treatment almost always is effective. The most frequent error in diagnosis is failure to consider the possibility of seizures as an explanation for aberrant behavior, whether or not other signs of central nervous system dysfunction are present.

The simplest all-inclusive definition of a *clinical seizure* is a paroxysmal, recurrent, stereotyped alteration of brain function. The exception to this definition is the occurrence of but a single convulsion, usually one associated with fever. Otherwise, no qualification is needed for the wide variety of clinical manifestations; neither convulsive movements nor loss of consciousness is necessary in seizure disorders. Recurrent episodes in which retention of consciousness is associated with complete absence of movement should make one suspicious of another process such as drug intoxication or one of the periodic paralyses.

Any unexplained behavior, particularly if it is episodic in nature, always warrants careful investigation for the possibility it may derive from a seizure state. In infancy and early childhood there are two types of behavior about which there should be a high degree of suspicion: staring episodes which do not respond to the visual obstruction of *holding* a hand in front of the child's eyes; and crying episodes which start abruptly for no apparent reason, cannot be assuaged no matter what is done, and terminate just as abruptly, with resumption of former activity.

Seizures occur in three different groups of individuals: those who have (1) seizures and other manifestations of organic brain disease, or (2) seizures alone, or (3) an apparent mental deficiency secondary to a seizure state.

In the first group, the seizures can be treated and controlled, with great benefit to the child and the family, but the accompanying disorders such as mental deficiency or "cerebral palsy" are not altered. When seizures are the only demonstrable evidence of central nervous system dysfunction, treatment is vital, episodes can be controlled and potential deterioration prevented, but the developmental rate is not necessarily accelerated. In the third group, the children appear to be mentally defective because they are out of contact as a result of their almost constant seizure activity. Although there is only a small number in this third category, treatment is rewarding, since it results in a "cure" of the seeming mental deficiency.

In the presence of uncontrolled seizures, no predictions regarding intellectual potential can be made until adequate therapy is instituted and the episodes abolished.

SENSORY IMPAIRMENT

COMMUNICATION DISORDERS

Communication with verbal symbols is one of man's most distinctive characteristics. Normal development of communication depends on the intactness of the mechanisms for hearing, language comprehension, and motor expression. Hearing is a specialized form of tactile sense which makes the organism aware of vibrations of distant origin and enables him to get into *touch* with what is spatially remote.

Hearing Impairment. Hearing includes both the perception of a sound stimulus and its interpretation by complex cortical and subcortical mechanisms.

Impairment of the mechanics of the external or middle ear produces a *conductive hearing loss,* with decrease in the ability to hear across all frequency ranges. Air conduction is impaired, while bone conduction is intact. Sound is muffled but not distorted. When medical or surgical intervention is not curative, sound amplification with a hearing aid results in normal ability to discriminate language except in unusual circumstances.

Sensorineural hearing loss poses an entirely different problem. This hearing loss is not symmetric but usually is greater at the higher frequencies. The child hears some of everything going on about her, but it is distorted; the necessary acoustic detail is missing, and discrimination and language comprehension are lost. The resultant handicap depends not only on the degree of the loss but on the frequencies at which the loss occurs. Mere amplification of all sound does not remedy the situation for her. Modern hearing aids can amplify sounds differentially across frequencies sufficiently to restore some balance and permit reasonable discrimination of the spoken word. However, when there is a loss of 70 decibels or more at all frequencies, sound amplification adequate for the development of good speech rarely can be accomplished. The term *deaf,* as contrasted with *hearing impaired,* now is reserved for this relatively small percentage of individuals.

Because of resistance to the concept of congenital aphasia, *central communication disorder* or *central auditory imperception* is used to describe those children who have no sensorineural hearing loss but nevertheless behave as though they were profoundly deaf. The terms are appropriate because the difficulty lies in the processing, patterning, and interpretation of the incoming sensory information within the brain. Sound often is so confusing that complete inhibition of response to all auditory stimuli results.

This type of auditory imperception occasionally may be an isolated phenomenon. In infants and preschool children, evidences of other impaired central nervous system function usually are easily detectable—disorganized behavior, neuromotor abnormalities, decreased response to visual and tactile cues, seizures, or varying degrees of intellectual impairment. Because both sensorineural and central communication hearing impairments can have common etiologic antecedents and common associated deficits, differential diagnosis may be difficult. However, it is very important to arrive at a diagnosis so that the child's training and education can be planned appropriately.

When there is a sensorineural hearing loss, sound amplification should be provided as early as possible—by 6–9 months of age. When the hearing impairment is of central origin, the approach to treatment is more controversial. The question is whether all sounds should be amplified, since auditory stimuli already are confusing, or whether auditory training should be restricted to specific situations geared to social communication. In contrast to those with sensorineural loss, most children with central communication disorders compensate eventually.

The cardinal objective in management of a child with hearing impairment is the conservation of all possible communication. *Socialization* to preserve the optimal growth of personality is a major goal.

Failure to Develop Speech. The most common reason for failure to develop *language* at the appropriate age is mental deficiency. Speech production is only one facet of language development. Often the clinician is faced with a 2- or 3-year-old who uses no words. Three things must then be determined by developmental assessment: Does the child have normal intelligence? Does she hear? Does she understand what is said to her? If the answers to these questions are "yes," the child will talk when what she wishes to communicate cannot be transmitted adequately by means of gesture and pantomime. The parents must avoid pressuring the child to talk and should emphasize intercommunication instead. Any congenital anomalies which could involve the motor mechanisms for producing sound would have become apparent before this age. Formal speech therapy for articulatory defects which might become manifest will be more effective if delayed to 4 or 4½ years of age.

VISUAL DISORDERS

Vision is the most sophisticated and objective of all the senses. It gives the most detailed report of the outside world by simultaneously registering position, distance, size, color, and form. But vision does not function in complete isolation; developmentally and psychologically it is closely correlated with other sensory activities, particularly touch and kinesthesia. From the very beginning there is a motor component in the infant's visual behavior. The retina receives impressions, and the muscles, fundamental and accessory, achieve adjustments to position, distance, size, and form. The cortex organizes the experience. Vision is more precocious than audition in its development, but both looking and listening are criteria of cortical intactness in the newborn period.

Visual Defect. The blind infant cannot attain even the most rudimentary spatial orientations until he can bring his muscular system to bear upon the problems of position, distance, size, and form. But for him they always will be different problems, because he cannot use sight and motor responses in mutual self-correcting combination and reciprocal reinforcement.

However, the blind child has a progressive ability to meet the basic tests of life if he is otherwise normal. Some of the child's failures and difficulties must be ascribed to his handicap, but too much allowance should not be made for the retarding effect of the blindness *per se*. If he has normal potentialities, he will demonstrate them in the total integration of his behavior. If his behavior is fragmentary and poorly organized or if it is extremely self-absorbed and undirected, the outlook is not promising. Blindness does not necessarily produce serious retardation.

However, blindness constitutes more than a mere absence or impairment of a single sense. If it dates from birth or early infancy, it may dislocate drastically the entire mental life of the child. For these reasons, the retention of even a very slight amount of vision in a visually defective infant has a favorable effect on his behavioral organization. Any therapeutic or surgical procedure in infancy which can bestow even a modicum of sight is paramount above other measures. Unfortunately, any primary or secondary damage to the visual receptors is extremely likely to involve other structures of the brain and may produce mental deficiency. The restoration of some vision does not always insure a favorable developmental outlook, even when accomplished early.

In the early education of the blind, confusion must be avoided. Ideally there should be a deliberate simplification of the world of sounds for the blind child. There should be fixed orientations with respect to rooms, playground, doors, and furniture. The dim world of the partially seeing should be earmarked by certain fixed sounds such as the chime of a clock and the ring of a bell. It should be eyemarked by conspicuous identification disks and by spotlights which draw attention to locations. When an adult is at hand to safeguard, the blind baby can be encouraged to creep and the toddler to walk.

Self-confidence can be imparted by progressive stages, with not too much reliance on the hard knocks of experience.

Visual Cortical Dysfunction. There is a group of children, analagous to those with central communication disorders, whose handicaps are due to cerebral impairment involving chiefly the visual areas. More than strabismus results; a serious visual impairment is the presenting symptom. These children often are referred for diagnosis as blind or near-blind. Vision is very defective but not altogether absent. The infant cocks his head to see, the eyes rove and he sees but fleetingly, "out of the corner of his eye." Often he will perceive only a moving object. When the defect is extreme, avoidance of very bright light or a pupillary response may be the only signs of an intact end organ.

At the same time, the child almost invariably shows evidences of associated impairment of motor function. These evidences may be only minimal, but it is very important that they be recognized. Any combination of visual and manual disabilities may distort and reduce adaptive behavior to a marked degree.

A great many of these children eventually learn to use what little vision they have with considerable effectiveness. However, the precise degree of effective vision cannot be predicted in infancy. Most of the children can walk about without guidance. Some compensate almsot completely by school age. The parents must learn to think of their child not in terms of his eyes but in terms of his total makeup, including his associated handicaps and assets. Prognosis for development depends on the normality of these assets and the intelligence of parental management.

QUALITATIVE AND INTEGRATIVE ASPECTS

Movement of some kind underlies virtually all behavior, so deviations in motor patterns are the most prominent feature of neurologic impairment in early life. However, they are not the only manifestations of central nervous system dysfunction. Three other aspects of behavior indicate the organization of the central nervous system characteristic for a particular individual (often referred to as "temperament"): attention, activity, and emotional stability.

Normally, when a stimulus is presented, an examiner literally can "see the wheels go round" and watch the infant or child perceive it and make an appropriate response. Appropriate responses can be distorted by extremes of environmental impoverishment, but the normal child is interested and stimulated by an examination situation. When integration is impaired, attention may be described as variable, fleeting, distractible and capricious or, alternatively, as perseverative and unduly fixated. Concomitantly, exploitation may be designated haphazard, impulsive, and disorganized or, in contrast, stereotyped. Rarely do these distortions appear in the absence of motor, sensory, intellectual, or convulsive manifestations. If they do, environmental causes should be sought.

The activity level of normal children varies widely, from the "sedentary intellectual" to the "athlete." Hyperactivity as a pathologic phenomenon occupies a place of prominence in current concern with behavioral aberration. The term requires very precise definition. The essential qualities of hyperactivity are its inappropriate, nondirected and irrelevant nature, and the inability of the child to control it. Hyperkinesis must be distinguished from gross motor drive, from normal motor activity bothersome to parents because of unduly high expectations for control, and from lack of appropriate play opportunities available to the child. Also, evaluation must be made in a structured and interesting situation in which the child is expected to "settle down." A diagnosis of hyperactivity should be reserved only for the individual who continues to show tangential responses in circumstances which normally elicit organized behavior.

Emotional stablility, or lack of it, is more difficult to evaluate as a manifestation of brain dysfunction because there are great individual differences. Some children make an immediate, sociable and absorbed response to the examiner and the examination. Others are fragile, labile, irritable, uninterested or tentative, and withdraw to their mothers. In the ordinary couse of events, even the initially suspicious child usually succumbs, and by the end of the session may permit the examiner to pick him up or perform a physical examination. Whether or not persistent emotional fragility in the absence of any other abnormalities indicates brain dysfunction, it certainly can interfere with adjustment to life situations.

Infantile Psychosis. One of the most serious disturbances of central nervous system function falls under this general heading. From a very early age, the normal infant is socially responsive to people. When the give and take of normal *social interaction* does not unfold, or is lost, the child's behavior seems to arise from within himself. It appears unrelated to environmental stimuli and is accompanied by a variety of repetitive bizarre mannerisms; there may be aggressive, destructive and self-destructive acts. Nowhere does more confusion exist than in this group of children, who currently are diagnosed as suffering from infantile psychoses, variously termed autism, childhood schizophrenia, atypical ego development, symbiotic psychosis or a heterogeneous group of other designations. They are frequently thought of as having psychogenic psychiatric disorders, and are so treated.

Clinical pictures of schizophrenia comparable to the adult disease, in children who have been essentially healthy, seldom develop before 8 years of age; they are seen with increasing frequency towards adolescence. There is consensus that the term *childhood schizophrenia* should be reserved for such previously healthy children, and *infantile psychosis* or *autism* employed for those in whom the picture has been present from birth or early life.

Consequently, the clearest picture of the antecedents and associated findings in autism is obtained when children are seen on a pediatric developmental disabilities service. Our experience on such a service indicates that autism is not a specific disease entity. Rather it is a description of a specific type of behavior in which the infant or child fails to regard people as persons. It is highly associated with prenatal and neonatal abnormalities and always associated with organic disease of the brain of some kind and degree. The concomitant diseases run the gamut of neuropsychiatric disabilities of congenital, infectious, traumatic, teratologic, and degenerative origin. Mental deficiency, which may be profound, is found in 75-80% of the children. Compensation occurs with maturation, and the persistence of the autistic behavior and ultimate functional ability depend on the degree of intellectual impairment, the nature of the associated conditions, and the adequacy of appropriate educational experiences.

SPECIFIC SYNDROMES

Dysmorphic physical features and biochemical abnormalities often are found associated with neuropsychiatric disabilities, especially with mental deficiency. Sometimes these are characteristic of specific hereditary diseases, of chromosomal disorders, inborn errors of metabolism or of other syndromes with a known predictable course. It is important to recognize these conditions. Some have implications for genetic counseling, others require specific therapy. In our experience, all trisomic chromosomal disorders sooner or later show deceleration in developmental rate.

6
Recording and Appraisal

A record which includes the following should be made of every assessment: a history; the developmental schedules; an evaluation of the quality of the behavior, intellectual potential, and neuromotor status; a diagnostic summary; and a written report of the assessment. Detailed forms for the history and the developmental and neurologic status, which are designed for computerization and a minimum of writing, appear in Appendix A-5 of Developmental Diagnosis. *They are available from the authors. The essential elements from them which should be incorporated in the records of any developmental disabilities service are discussed and listed in the following sections. Reference to the complete forms will clarify some of the briefer listings included here. Appropriate identifying information should, of course, be part of any form.*

HISTORY

Historic information is acquired by two methods, and ideally should be obtained before proceeding to the examination. The appropriate Revised Parent Developmental Questionnaire is mailed to the parents prior to their appointment in order to obtain information about the child's developmental progress. This questionnaire is reproduced and discussed in Chapter 7. The parents' answers to these questions are transferred to the corresponding items on the developmental schedules.

When the parents bring their child for his assessment, a history form is completed. The information obtained should be recorded directly on the form as it is elicited from the parents. Finally, additional items of behavior and any necessary clarification of the parents' responses to the questionnaire are recorded directly on the appropriate developmental schedules as they are being obtained.

The history should be recorded and should include the information shown in the following sample.

Date of Birth __1/1/78__

Chief Complaint __Were told he is mongoloid, but he's doing so well!__

Family History:

Father's Age, Education, Occupation __41, 12, plumber__

Mother's Age, Education, Occupation __39, 12, housewife__

Parity Sequence __53114; 15-year-old with hare lip; 12N; miscarriage; 10N__

Any Central Nervous System Disease __None__

Other Hereditary Disease __None__

Present Pregnancy:

Birth Weight __2495 grams__

Expected Date of Confinement __1/15/78__

Gestational Age __38 weeks__

Corrected Birth Date if Indicated __1/15/78__

Toxemia __None__

Spotting __At first missed period__

Bleeding __Moderate, after membranes ruptured__

Chronic Disease __None__

Acute Illnesses __None__

Medication, Drugs __Vitamins__

Neonatal Course:

Days in Hospital __6__

Respiratory Difficulty __Stopped breathing once; oxygen 2 days__

Seizure Activity __None__

Feeding Difficulty _None_

Jaundice _None_

Illnesses _None_

Subsequent Course:

Feeding Difficulty _None_

Muscle Tone Changes _None until 4 months; right leg a little stiff_

Acute Illnesses or Accidents _Roseola at 4 months_

Chronic Diseases _None_

Congenital Anomalies _Mongoloid; slight heart disease_

Vision or Hearing Problems _None_

Seizures _Grand Mal, ½ hour long, with roseola; no treatment_

Has Child Ever Failed to Make Progress _No_

Has Child Ever Lost
      Behavior Once Achieved _Didn't use right arm and leg as well after convulsion_

Age at First Concern About Child's Development _Birth–chromosomes abnormal_

Is There a Normal Social Give-and-Take ("Autism") _Yes_

Behavior Problems _None_

Parental Disagreements About Child _None_

DEVELOPMENTAL SCHEDULES

Several possible methods of recording an examination are noted in Chapter 2. Videotape is the best. Even brief notes made by the examiner during the course of the examination are apt to disturb the flow of a child's behavior. It is far better if he can train himself to retain a vivid memory picture of what the child does and record it on the forms immediately after the examination, adding descriptive notes and comments.

No matter how the examination is recorded, the child's performance always is noted first on the developmental schedules. The examiner makes use of his clinical impression of the child in selecting
(Text continued on p 174)

Excerpt from Revised Gesell Developmental Schedule

Name: *John Doe* CC Age: *28 weeks* Date *7/28/78* Case *#0001*

24 Weeks

H	O	ADAPTIVE
+	N	Ra: 2-hand approach & grasp (*28w)
	+	Ra: shakes actively
+	+	Ra: reaches after dropped rattle
	N	Cube: 2-hand approach & grasp (*28w)
+	±	Cube, Bell: to mouth
	+	Cubes: resecures dropped cube
	+	M. Cubes: grasps 1st, grasps 2nd
	+	M. Cubes: exploits 3 cubes
+	+	Cup & M. Cubes: retains cube, regards cup (*28w)
	-	Yarn: looks for fallen yarn

H	O	GROSS MOTOR
-	-	Supine: lifts head from platform
+	+	Supine: rolls to prone
-	-	Pull-to-Sit: lifts head, assists (*36w)
+	+	Chair: trunk erect (*36w)
░	±	Sit: well, leaning on hands (*28w)
-	-	Stand: bounces (*28w) (*supports weight*)

KEY AGE 28 Weeks

H	O	ADAPTIVE	
+	+	Cube, Bell: 1-hand approach & grasp	25(23-27)
	-	2nd Cube: grasps 1st, grasps 2nd	
	░	2nd Cube: grasps 2 more than momentarily	
	░	3rd Cube: retains 2 as 3rd presented	
	+	Massed Cubes: grasps 2 more than momentarily	
	+	Cup & Massed Cubes: retains cube, grasps cup	
+	±	Cube, Bell, Ring-String: transfers cube adeptly (*awkward*)	
+	+	Cube, Bell, Ring-String: bangs	
	-	Bell: retains (*? disability*)	
	░	Ring-String: secures ring by string (*40w)	

H	O	GROSS MOTOR	
	-	Sit: sits erect about 1 minute	22
	-	Stand: stands hands held (*32w)	
	-	Prone: pivots (*36w)	
	-	Prone: assumes creeping position	
	-	Prone: crawls or creep-crawls (*36w)	

	FINE MOTOR			FINE MOTOR	
	± Cube: palmar grasp (*28w)(L > R)		▓	− Cube: radial palmar grasp (*36w)	24
	+ Pellet: contacts, rakes with whole hand (*28w)			− Pellet: radial raking or unsuccessful inferior scissors grasp (*32w)	
	+ String: contacts, rakes with whole hand (*28w)			− String: inferior scissors grasp (*40w)	
	LANGUAGE			**LANGUAGE**	
	+ Bird Call, Bell-Ring: turns head		−	− Vocalization: ah-ah-ah, oh-oh-oh, not aaah (*32w)	25
+	Expressive: displeasure by sound other than crying (*——)		+	+ Vocalization: mum-mum-mum, crying (*36w)	
			−	− Vocalization: single consonant sounds—da, ba, ga	
			−	− Vocalization: imitates sounds—cough, tongue-click, razz	
	PERSONAL-SOCIAL			**PERSONAL-SOCIAL**	
−	Feeding: takes solids well		+	+ Play: feet to mouth	26
+	Social: creates social contact		−	− Play: persistent for toys out of reach	
+	Social: pushes mother's hand away (*——)		+	+ Play: bites & chews	
+	Play: grasps feet, supine				
+	Play: sits propped 30 minutes (*36w)				
+	Mirror: pats mirror image				

H = History; O = Observation   (*) = pattern replaced by more mature one at later age the appropriate developmental schedule(s) for recording. He selects the schedules in terms of key ages and says to himself, "This child is viewed best in terms of 16 weeks—or 40 weeks—or 2 years," whatever the case may be.

On all developmental schedules, two columns are provided: H for history, and O for observation. The use of both history and observation columns allows the examiner to indicate that the information given by the parent has been confirmed. Some information is available only by report, particularly in language and personal-social behavior. In instances of disagreement, the parents' report is accepted and the observation column left blank unless the examiner observes the pattern which was reported as lacking. A pattern is recorded as lacking in the face of a positive report only when there is overwhelming evidence that the parents' information is inaccurate. As already indicated in Chapter 2, rejection of parental information is a very risky venture.

In recording observed behavior on the chosen schedule(s), the examiner must remember that there are two types of behavior patterns: *permanent* patterns and *temporary* patterns. Temporary patterns are ones which are transformed or are replaced by different and more advanced patterns at later stages. Temporary patterns are indicated on the schedules by an asterisk; the age at which the pattern is replaced by a more advanced pattern also is given. Some temporary patterns form part of a sequence; an infant cannot sit indefinitely without first being able to sit for 10 minutes, or hold his head at a 90° but not a 45° angle while prone. Other temporary patterns are completely replaced by more mature patterns; the scissors grasp of 36 weeks is replaced by the inferior princer grasp at 40 weeks. In a transitional phase, both may be seen. In addition to knowing whether the less mature pattern has been discarded completely, we wish to indicate if any particular item is an integral part of the child's behavior or merely incipient.

To record these complexities in observed behavior patterns adequately, the following code is provided:

A *plus sign* (+) is entered when any behavior pattern on the schedule is well-established as an organic part of the child's working equipment. If a behavior pattern is accomplished in a "singles" situation, a positive response can be assumed in its comparable "multiple" situation. For example, grasps 2 cubes prolongedly at 32 and 28 weeks, respectively. If copying or naming is accomplished, that behavior clearly supersedes the comparable imitating or pointing.

A *plus-minus* (±) is entered for a pattern that is incidental or incipient, but not yet fully integrated. It also indicates situations where a response is intermediate, for example, puts 7 cubes into cup rather than 9 at 56 weeks. Circling this designation prevents confusion with adjacent entries. At times both a temporary pattern and its replacement are present, and both receive a plus (+) sign. However, when a behavior pattern on the schedule is not represented in the child's repertoire, the examiner must pause.

A *minus sign* (−) is entered when a permanent pattern (no asterisk) is not part of the child's behavior *or* when a lacking temporary pattern (asterisk) has not yet been superseded by its more mature pattern.

When a temporary pattern is lacking because the child is displaying more advanced superseding behavior instead, there are two possibilities:

A *double plus sign* (++) is used when the behavior is part of an obligatory sequence, *e.g.*, sits 10 min⁺ *and* steadily at 32 and 36 weeks.

N (no longer necessary) is employed when the temporary pattern has been replaced entirely by the more mature pattern with which it is mutually exclusive, *e.g.*, scissors grasp replaced by inferior pincer.

While the distinction between ++ and *N* may seem needlessly complicated, it does serve the examiner by emphasizing visually the developmental progressions and indicating clearly when the less mature pattern has been discarded completely. For computer analysis, when only individual items are examined and no total picture is in view, the nature of any given pattern is delineated more clearly by this device.

In summary, a + or ± sign entered for any pattern on the schedule means that the child displayed the pattern; a ++ or *N* sign means he displayed a more mature pattern instead; a − sign means that he is not yet mature enough with respect to that particular pattern to display it. *By this device we preserve the fundamental connotation of the minus sign.*

Other notations can be placed to the left of the history column to help add qualitative dimensions to the observed behavior.

A *(abnormal)* denotes that a pattern is present or incipient but abnormal in its expression.

D (*disability*) is entered if some adaptive or language item of behavior is not accomplished because of a motor or sensory handicap (*e.g.*, no transfer in an infant with hemiplegia, or no words in a child with hearing impairment). It may also accompany a + sign to indicate that assistance is needed or some other variation occurs. For example, an infant is unable to pick up a pellet, at 36 weeks, no matter how hard she tries; when she holds the bottle she is as persistent for the pellet as she was for the pellet alone. *D* should not be entered for a motor behavior pattern; absence in itself constitutes disability. It rarely is possible to differentiate disability from immaturity when an item is just appearing at the child's chronologic age (*e.g.*, the 28-week-old who does not grasp the second cube, or the 56-week-old who does not build a tower of two cubes).

R (*refusal*) can be used when the child refuses a situation, usually at the very beginning of the examination before she has adjusted, or for gross motor activity. *R should not* be substituted for a minus (−) sign when the child's behavior indicates that her typical reaction is to reject actively tasks she perceives as too difficult for her.

There is one further general principle to be followed. When recording performance in an area of behavior for any given age, enter some notation for every pattern in that specific area (other areas at that age may be completely blank). When you review the record at a later date, you will have no idea why there is a blank if you fail to take this simple precaution.

X indicates there is no information about a particular area because you deliberately or inadvertently omitted it, or no history was available.

? indicates that you don't remember or can't interpret what the infant did.

For the novice's encouragement, it may be added that when there is familiarity with developmental sequences, and with a little practice, recording becomes faster and almost automatic.

To recapitulate:

1. On the basis of history and observations, the examiner selects the developmental schedule containing the most appropriate Key Age for recording.
2. He enters a + or ± sign whenever the child demonstrates the behavior pattern.
3. He enters a + + or *N* sign whenever the child fails to display a

temporary pattern *because the child displayed a more mature pattern instead.*

4. He enters a − sign whenever the child fails to display a permanent pattern, or whenever he fails to display a temporary pattern *because he displayed less mature patterns instead.*

5. He enters qualifying notations or comments and indicates missing information.

The examiner now is ready to appraise the child's maturity level in each area of behavior. The developmental schedule is used to list the presence and absence of significant behavior. We prefer to say "presence and absence" rather than "success or failure" because fundamentally we are concerned with status and not with success. There are no right or wrong responses; *any response is appropriate to some age level.* When we list the presence and absence of behavior patterns, we do not censor the child's behavior, we judge it.

From the standpoint of developmental diagnosis, the significance of plus and minus signs is always relative rather than absolute. The final estimate of developmental maturity is based on the *distribution* of plus and minus signs. *We do not sum and average the signs; it is the total clinical picture which is significant.* Maturity is appraised by determining how well a child's behavior fits one age level constellation rather than another. *In any field of behavior, the child's maturity level is that point where the aggregate of + signs changes to an aggregate of − signs.* For example, if a 40-week-old has all + signs in adaptive behavior at 40 weeks, removes the paper to uncover the cube and approaches the pellet first at 44 weeks, and tries to build a tower of 2 cubes at 48 weeks, an age level of 42 weeks would approximate most closely the adaptive maturity level. Thus, interpolation between adjacent levels is done, since a 40-week-old infant adds behavior gradually in achieving the next 44-week level of development. The assignment of the specific developmental age between 2 adjacent levels on the developmental schedule depends on which positive and negative patterns are present.

The plus and minus signs may be so irregularly distributed for a behavior area that this point of change becomes a band or zone of change, and no single age level can be determined. When this occurs, there are two possible ways of indicating it: a notation such as 35(26–38) denotes scatter and gaps but centering closer to the upper end of the range; 31(26–38) indicates the reverse. At times the behavior is so discrepant that the only adequate description is the range 26–38.

On occasion, only minimal information is available for any given area; the parents may not be available to provide a history of language or personal-social behavior, or the infant may be too ill or too inhibited to participate fully. For a 40-week infant, a notation such as 38-minimum would mean that the behavior is at least at the 38-week level, but the examiner feels that the optimum abilities have not been elicited. Such a notation is logical only when the behavior is in the normal range for the age of the child. For example, little information would be contributed to the assessment of the language behavior of a 40-week infant to record 26-minimum because you observed all of the 24-week behavior and heard single consonant sounds. In such circumstances no maturity level should be assigned.

A general developmental level is assigned which represents the intellectual potential. It is *not an average* of all 5 areas of behavior and is *never less than the adaptive level*. The adaptive level may be raised 1 or 2 weeks on the basis of good quality, the presence of interfering motor handicaps not already taken into consideration, or acceleration in language development. No general developmental level is assigned when language development is significantly more advanced than an adaptive level in the defective range. In such circumstances, there is obvious disorganization of behavior which requires further observation and investigation; language may be a better prognosticator of future potential than adaptive behavior.

The maturity levels assigned for each of the 5 areas and for the general developmental level can be noted in the margins on the developmental schedules and transferred later to a recording form. The maturity levels are the starting points for differential diagnosis, and their final interpretation is not made until the qualitative aspects of the behavior and neuromotor patterns are recorded and appraised.

DEVELOPMENTAL AND NEUROLOGIC EVALUATION

An evaluation of the quality of behavior, the intellectual potential, and the neuromotor status is the basis for the formulation of a diagnosis and prognosis, and for the subsequent interview with the parents to discuss them. Recording of abnormalities does not by itself explain them, however, and there must be a synthesis in a final report. The following minimal information should be gathered.

Qualitative Aspects of Behavior. If only the chronologic age of the child were taken into consideration in evaluating the quality of behavior, all children with mental deficiency would be markedly below average. No distinction could be made between those infants who showed behavior that was reasonably well-integrated for the age level at which they were functioning and those with varying degrees of disorganization associated with their mental defect. Consequently, a 40-week old with adaptive behavior of 24 weeks must be viewed in terms of responses appropriate to 24 weeks. He is abnormal, but *how* he responds to situations has an important bearing on his utilization of his potentialities, just as it does for a child with normal intelligence.

Quality of Integration: Note whether the behavior is above average, average, below average, or markedly below average.

Emotional Stability __*Average*__

Spontaneity __*Average*__

Rapport __*Average*__

Organization __*Below average*__

Attention __*Below average*__

Interest __*Below average*__

Maturity __*Average*__

Discrimination __*Average*__

Judgment __*Average*__

Exploitation __*Average*__

General Adjustment __*Average*__

Abnormal Behavior Patterns: Note whether the behavior is absent or normal in amount; or abnormal to mild, moderate, or marked degrees.

Perseveration __*Absent*__

Irritability __*Absent*__

Restlessness __*Mild*__

Hyperactivity _Mild_

Crying _Absent_

Stereotyped Mannerisms _Absent_

Scatter in Adaptive Behavior _Mild_

Dependency on Mother _Absent_

Muscle Tone and Movement. The same 40-week infant just referred to might have gross motor behavior which also is at the 24-week level. In terms of 40 weeks, one might be tempted to say she is hypotonic because of failure to sit and bear weight well. She *is* abnormal, but her muscle tone is appropriate for 24 weeks. In contrast, if gross motor behavior were 12 weeks, associated with decreased resistance to passive motion and decreased spontaneous activity, she would be hypotonic, in addition to having mental deficiency.

Hypotonicity must be evaluated in terms of the adaptive maturity level of the child. The other abnormalities in muscle tone and movement are qualitative changes which are abnormal at any age.

Note the presence or absence of the abnormality, and its degree and location.

Hypotonicity _Mild, left side and trunk_

Hypertonicity _None_

Spasticity _Mild, right side_

Dyskinesia
- Athetosis _None_
- Dystonia _None_
- Rigidity _None_

Ataxia _None_

Tremor _None_

Flaccidity _None_

Deep Tendon Reflexes _Increased, right leg_

Sensation: Note any hyper- or hypersthesia, the location and the level.
Normal

Special Sensory: Note the presence or absence of abnormality and its degree.

_____*None*_____

Vision:

Strabismus ___*Moderate alternating*_____

Nystagmus ___*None*_____

Ptosis ___*None*_____

Failure of Fixation ___*None*_____

Ocular Tilt, Peripheral Vision ___*None*_____

Visual Field Defect ___*None*_____

Fundi ___*Normal*_____

Visual Acuity ___*Normal*_____

Cortical Blindness ___*None*_____

Other ___*None*_____

Hearing:

Conductive Loss ___*None*_____

Sensorineural Loss ___*None*_____

Central Communication Disorder ___*None*_____

Infant Neuromotor Abnormalities. Whether a neuromotor pattern is abnormal depends on the age of the infant. It is not possible to make a list and apply all items at all ages. It is not abnormal for a 16-week old to have a rounded back in sitting or a 28-week old to have a whole-hand grasp; these are immature patterns which are appropriate for the respective chronologic ages. Further, there may be mental deficiency with retarded motor development but no other distortion of motor integration. The 40-week old discussed above *is* abnormal because of his mental deficiency, but his 24-week-old motor behavior may show that there are no abnormal neuromotor patterns for his 24-week level of function. A 2-year old with adaptive behavior at 11 months is not ataxic if he does not walk alone; he requires time, not referral to a cerebral palsy treatment center, to achieve independent locomotion.

Neuromotor patterns, whether normal or abnormal, must be considered in terms of the adaptive maturity age level of the infant, and the first step in their evaluation is the selection of the appropriate *adaptive* age zone.

16-week zone (15–23 weeks): Items bracketed with 3 asterisks ***; the rest are disregarded.

28-week zone (24–34 weeks): Items bracketed with 2 asterisks **; attention paid to *** and **, the rest are disregarded.

40-week zone (35 weeks+): Items bracketed with 1 asterisk *; all infant items are applicable above this age.

Children (when independent locomotion is attained; usually 56 weeks)

For example, for a 28-week zone, the degree of abnormality and whether it is unilateral or bilateral is noted for all items bracketed with 3 asterisks *and* with 2 asterisks.

Head:

Retraction	*None*
Backward Sagging	*Mild*
Forward Sagging	*None*
Sideward Sagging	*None*

Supine:

*
*
*

Persistent Tonic-Neck-Reflex	*None*
Extension of Legs	*None*
Scissoring	*None*

Sitting:

Persistent Tonic-Neck-Reflex	*None*
Extension of Legs	*Mild left, moderate right*
Narrow Base with Leg Adduction	*Mild left, moderate right*
Flexion of Knees and Hips	*Mild left, moderate right*

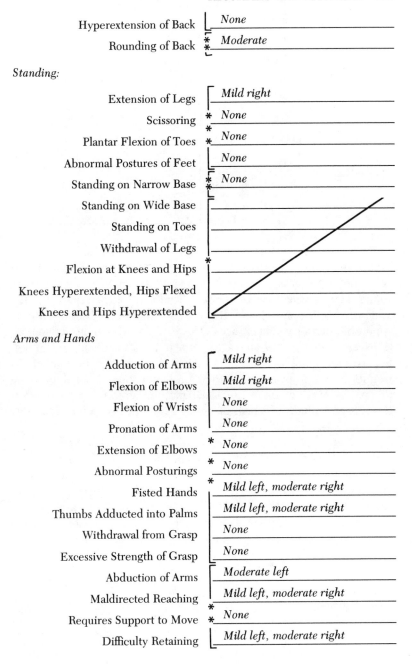

Hyperextension of Back — *None*

Rounding of Back — *Moderate*

Standing:

Extension of Legs — *Mild right*

Scissoring — *None*

Plantar Flexion of Toes — *None*

Abnormal Postures of Feet — *None*

Standing on Narrow Base — *None*

Standing on Wide Base

Standing on Toes

Withdrawal of Legs

Flexion at Knees and Hips

Knees Hyperextended, Hips Flexed

Knees and Hips Hyperextended

Arms and Hands

Adduction of Arms — *Mild right*

Flexion of Elbows — *Mild right*

Flexion of Wrists — *None*

Pronation of Arms — *None*

Extension of Elbows — *None*

Abnormal Posturings — *None*

Fisted Hands — *Mild left, moderate right*

Thumbs Adducted into Palms — *Mild left, moderate right*

Withdrawal from Grasp — *None*

Excessive Strength of Grasp — *None*

Abduction of Arms — *Moderate left*

Maldirected Reaching — *Mild left, moderate right*

Requires Support to Move — *None*

Difficulty Retaining — *Mild left, moderate right*

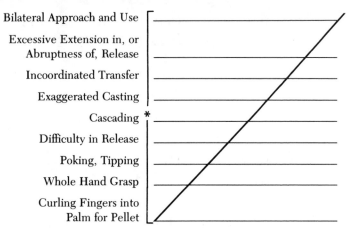

Bilateral Approach and Use
Excessive Extension in, or Abruptness of, Release
Incoordinated Transfer
Exaggerated Casting
Cascading *
Difficulty in Release
Poking, Tipping
Whole Hand Grasp
Curling Fingers into Palm for Pellet

Caution must be used in the interpretation of the infant neuromotor patterns prior to 16 weeks of age. Obviously, the very young infant normally has imperfect head control, persistence of the tonic-neck-reflex and fisted hands, and the form is not entirely applicable at the youngest ages. However, certain neuromotor patterns are abnormal at any age: retraction of the head, scissoring, hyperextension of the back, persistent flexion or extension of extremities (except for legs in sitting), and adduction of the thumb into the palm. Most of these abnormal patterns are present whenever there is a qualitative change in movement control, such as spasticity or dyskinesia.

Patterns in Children. Once independent locomotion has been attained, the infant patterns should be crossed out and any abnormalities recorded under the patterns for children. However, an older child with adaptive behavior above 56 weeks, but with a significant motor handicap, may have abnormal patterns at some or all of the infant levels, as well as in the patterns for children.

Lower Extremities:

Walking on Wide Base
Hyperextension of Knees

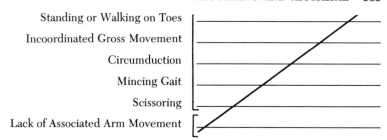

Standing or Walking on Toes
Incoordinated Gross Movement
Circumduction
Mincing Gait
Scissoring
Lack of Associated Arm Movement

Arms and Hands:

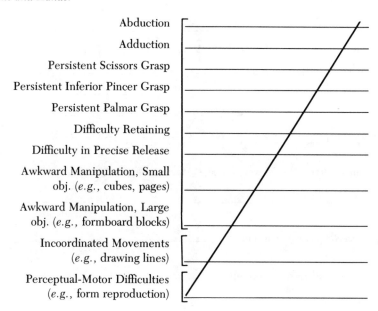

Abduction
Adduction
Persistent Scissors Grasp
Persistent Inferior Pincer Grasp
Persistent Palmar Grasp
Difficulty Retaining
Difficulty in Precise Release
Awkward Manipulation, Small obj. (*e.g.*, cubes, pages)
Awkward Manipulation, Large obj. (*e.g.*, formboard blocks)
Incoordinated Movements (*e.g.*, drawing lines)
Perceptual-Motor Difficulties (*e.g.*, form reproduction)

Speech (For Adaptive Age):

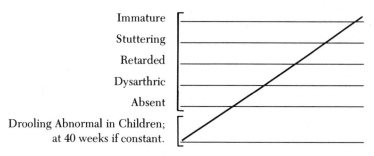

Immature
Stuttering
Retarded
Dysarthric
Absent
Drooling Abnormal in Children; at 40 weeks if constant.

Lack of associated arm movements and incoordinated movements in drawing lines are not abnormal until 24 months of age; perceptual-motor difficulties in form reproduction are not abnormal until 30 months.

The following additional information should be recorded for all children:

Substitutive Patterns: alternative methods utilized to overcome handicaps.

Reaches with Mouth _____*Mild*_____

Progresses by Rolling _____*None*_____

Arches while Supine, Using Feet _____*None*_____

Hitches in Sitting _____*None*_____

Crawls, Dragging Legs _____*None*_____

Casting or Cascading Instead of Grasping _____*None*_____

Poking or Tipping Instead of Grasping _____*None*_____

Locomotion: after 28 weeks of age. May be Retarded or Abnormal.

_____*Mild Retardation*_____

Miscellaneous Abnormalities: _____*None*_____

Observed Seizures: (Describe)

Abortive Grand Mal _____*None*_____

Psychomotor _____*None*_____

Myoclonic _____*None*_____

Grand Mal _____*None*_____

Petit Mal _____*None*_____

Other _____*None*_____

Autistic Behavior: _____*None*_____

Physical Defects (Other than Neurologic): May be Minor, Major, or Temporary

_____*Small VSD, no limitation of activity*_____

Estimate of Mother's Handling of Child: (Circle).

(Relaxed) (Self-assured) Tense   Uncertain   Unperceptive
Other _____

DEVELOPMENTAL QUOTIENTS (DQ)

The maturity age levels assigned on the developmental schedules are transferred to the form and are the basis for calculating developmental quotients.

$$DQ = \frac{\text{Maturity Age}}{\text{Chronologic Age}} \times 100$$

DQ	Maturity Age (Weeks or Months)	
089	25 (23–27)	General Developmental Level
089	25 (23–27)	Adaptive Behavior
079	22	Gross Motor Behavior
086	24	Fine Motor Behavior
089	25	Language Behavior
093	26	Personal-Social Behavior

SYNTHESIS

The examiner is ready now to summarize and appraise the child's total behavior and formulate diagnosis and prognosis. In appraising maturity, the examiner also must undertake to explain, or at least give weight to, discrepancies—behavior patterns seriously out of line with the child's total picture. He must take into account factors that might influence the behavioral responses: illness, fatigue, apprehension, insecurity, unhappiness, visual and hearing defects, motor handicaps, seizures, or language difficulties. The child always is interpreted in terms of his age, his experiences, his capabilities, and his environment. A penetrating appraisal of this kind tells much more than the child's maturity status; it sums up his characteristics, the integrity of his organization, and his latent and realized potentialities.

Intellectual Potential: Adequacy of Examination for Prediction. A statement that the examination is adequately predictive assumes that the environment and subsequent educational opportunities will be optimum, or at least satisfactory. For a normal infant, the precise IQ attained at school age will depend on the sociocultural status of the parents. Later experience will affect the function of a child with mental deficiency also, but an enriched environment will not make him normal. A statement that the examination is indicative of present function, but that modifying factors are present, implies that the behavior elicited is fairly typical and that the child has exhibited this to the best of his ability, but that a diagnosis or a firm prognosis for the future cannot be given. A child who has spent his life in an institution can improve after placement in a good foster home. An infant with frequent seizures may appear grossly defective but show a few fragments of age-appropriate behavior; he may function entirely normally when his seizures are controlled. A severe motor handicap may interfere with exploitation, but attention and interest may be maintained for an hour or more. Conversely, an infant with trisomy 21 may have normal adaptive behavior at 6 months of age, but deceleration and subsequent mental deficiency of some degree are the rule. A statement that the examination is inadequate for precise evaluation means that the child was not participating fully. Enough behavior may be elicited to indicate that mental deficiency is not present, but a precise maturity level representing optimum performance cannot be determined. In rare instances (less than 1%) the child simply refuses to cooperate, the examination is entirely inadequate and few or no details of any kind can be recorded.

Note the applicable characterization.

Adequate _____

Indicative of Present Function
    but Modifying Factors Present __*Trisomy 21, expect deceleration*__

Inadequate for Precise Evaluation _____

Inadequate _____

Intellectual Potential: Clinical Evaluation. The clinical evaluation of intellectual potential is a qualitative description of the performance which obviously is related to the general adaptive developmental quotient, but is not rigidly defined by the numerical value calculated.

Marked acceleration in itself does not indicate superiority; conversely, moderate acceleration combined with unusual maturity and novel exploitation might be so designated. A decision between dull normal and borderline dull is made on the basis of the quality and integration of the behavior. The category "indeterminate, not defective," usually is employed when the examination is inadequate for precise evaluation but behavior is in the normal range. "Undecided" generally indicates that behavior is qualitatively abnormal but the extent of the mental deficiency is in doubt.

In Normal Range	*Mental Deficiency Present or Likely*
____ Superior	____ Borderline Dull
____ High Average	____ Borderline Defective
____ Average	____ Defective, mild
✔ Low Average	____ Defective, moderate
____ Dull Normal	____ Defective, severe
____ Indeterminate, not defective	____ Undecided

Neuromotor Status. Neuromotor status is concerned with posture, locomotion, movement control, muscle tone, coordination, manipulation, and reflexes. The examiner makes her diagnosis of neuromotor status on the basis of both the maturity level of the child and the abnormal patterns recorded. If she determines that some neuromotor disorganization is present, she must decide on its nature and degree. The definitions of the various degrees of abnormality are delineated in Chapter 5. When the intellectual potential has been recorded as Normal, the neuromotor status is indicated in the 1st section below under degree of abnormality. When mental deficiency is present or likely, neuromotor status is recorded in the 2nd section. A diagnosis of abnormal signs of severe degree, with qualitative changes in movement control, is independent of the intellectual potential.

Type of Neuromotor Abnormality:

No Abnormality _____

Disease Outside Central Nervous System _____

Chronic Organic Brain Disease __✔_____

Other Central Nervous System Disease _____

Multiple Conditions _____

Degree of Neuromotor Abnormality:

1. Intellectual Potential Normal:

   No Abnormality _____

   Abnormal Signs of No Clinical Importance _____

   Abnormal Signs of Minor Degree _____

   Abnormal Signs of Marked Degree _____

2. Mental Deficiency Present or Likely:

   Normal for Chronologic Age _____

   Motor Retardation with:
   No Abnormal Signs for Level _____

   Abnormal Signs of No Clinical Importance _____

   Abnormal Signs of Minor Degree _____

   Abnormal Signs of Marked Degree _____

3. Abnormal Signs of Severe Degree:

   Qualitative Change in Movement Control: ___*Mild right spastic hemiplegia*___

Qualitative Aspects. A summary of the emotional stability and quality of integration permits the examiner to indicate at least two of the most important possible explanations for abnormalities in behavior. Seizures may affect the behavior continuously or intermittently. An "autistic" child may have well-organized exploitation of the test objects in the absence of an awareness of people.

As indicated previously, the qualitative aspects must be considered in relation to the adaptive maturity of the child. Note whether there are mild, moderate or severe disturbances and whether seizures or "autism" is present.

Emotional Stability ___*Normal*___

Quality of Integration ___*Mild disorganization*___

Seizures; "autism;" both ___*None*___

Neuromotor Potential. The neuromotor potential is summarized in terms of what is to be expected when a standard neurologic examination is done at school age. *Normal* includes those children with no neuromotor abnormality and those with abnormal signs of no clinical importance. Those children with abnormal signs of minor or marked degree, with the hypotonic type of "cerebral palsy," or with other clinical conditions in which recovery or gross compensation is anticipated, would be expected to have *No Significant Neuromotor Sequelae.* If some degree of *Abnormality* would be detected by the classical neurologic examination, *make an estimate of the degree of severity.*

Neuromotor Potential ___*Minimal right-sided involvement*___

Total Potential Other Than Physical. The major factor influencing the potential other than physical is the child's intelligence, which presupposes no subsequent noxious events. The infant with "autism" usually compensates; seizures are treatable. "Below average" is used for the clinical designation of dull normal, borderline dull or borderline defective, and "markedly below average" when a definite diagnosis of mental deficiency is anticipated.

Potential Other Than Physical ___*Markedly below average*___

Diagnostic Summary. As a final step, a brief notation is made in each of the 6 major areas in the Diagnostic Summary. Although it is completed last, a position of prominence on the first page of any form provides a quick overview when the chart is perused later.

Intellectual ___*Low average at present*___
Neuromotor ___*Mild right spastic hemiplegia*___
Seizures ___*Grand Mal (at 4 months)*___
Special Sensory ___*None*___
Qualitative ___*Mild disorganization*___
Specific Diseases or Syndromes ___*Trisomy 21*___

If the infant is essentially normal, the experienced clinician might elect to omit a detailed form, and instead make a few descriptive notes on the back of the developmental schedule before writing a final report. Less skilled examiners always should complete an entire form.

In this way they will incorporate observation and interpretation of any possible abnormalities as an integral and routine part of their examination procedure.

FINAL REPORT OF THE EVALUATION

The appended format was evolved as a guide for students, house staff, and fellows. The purposes of a report are to clarify what has been heard and observed, to give the data on which diagnosis, prognosis, and recommendations for treatment are based, and to transmit this information in a clear and understandable way to others. Certain basic information is included for all children, but the report is geared toward a specific description of the distinctive abilities and disabilities of the child under consideration.

    I. Identifying information:
       Record patient's name, case number, birth date, age (or corrected chronologic age), person to whom original copy of report goes, and persons to receive carbon copies.

   II. Reason for examination.

  III. History (use past tense):
      A. Birth weight and duration of gestation: Note if amount of prematurity was assigned arbitrarily because of discrepancies between history of gestation and birth weight, and reason for making adjustments.
      B. Pregnancy, labor and delivery, and neonatal period: Mention abnormalities specifically associated with high risk.
      C. Significant illnesses.
      D. Convulsions: Type of episodes, age of onset, frequency, duration, association with fever, and treatment.
      E. Developmental history: Indicate if normal or in what areas significant deviation occurred, and age at which deviation first was noted. Note specifically if deterioration has occurred.

  IV. Qualitative description of behavior (use present tense for remainder):
      Mention specific patterns which characterize the behavior of this child, as well as any physical anomalies that will call him to mind. Include both unusual distortions in sequences (*e.g.,*

exploits on touch rather than on visual perception) or outstandingly mature patterns. Comments on general description, adjustment to the examination, interest and attention, and quality of exploitation are included as a rule.

V. Neuromotor abnormalities:

  A. Abnormal patterns appropriate for the child's functional age are described. Some will warrant description in the examiner's own words, being specific rather than general, e.g., "shows incoordination in use of a pencil in drawing," rather than merely "incoordinated movements."

  B. Describe any seizures observed during the examination.

  C. Where speech development is a problem, comment on the comprehension of language as well.

  D. Mention visual or auditory deficits.

  E. If there are no significant neuromotor abnormalities, a sentence to this effect at end of paragraph IV is sufficient.

VI. Behavior characteristics (do not use "he is able to . . ."):

  Each area of the developmental schedules is taken separately, in order. Within each area, give observed items first, then reported behavior. Group together related behavior, e.g., cube, pellet, supine, prone. Not all items necessarily are included, and negatives are mentioned only if they are particularly pertinent to the problem. Do not include the less mature item of a sequence if a more advanced one is positive, e.g., omit "stands and supports large fraction of his weight" (20 weeks) if infant also stands with hands held (28 weeks). The assigned maturity level for each area is placed in parentheses after each field subheading.

VII. Diagnosis:

  A. The following three items are detailed first: The general maturity level, the quality of the behavior, and the level of development indicated. If development is average, include only a qualitative statement, such as high average or average. If it is not average, give the percentage of normal development, followed by a qualitative phrase, e.g., "Maturity is 55–60% of normal and a mild degree of mental deficiency is indicated."

  B. Do not list maturity levels in all areas of behavior in the diagnostic paragraph. Unless there is an indication, such as is specified below, other areas are not mentioned.

C. Gross motor behavior is mentioned specifically if it has diagnostic importance, *e.g.*, "Gross motor behavior is approximately X weeks, and John has 'cerebral palsy,' which is an athetoid quadriplegia." Give the neuromotor diagnosis when it is abnormal. For normal infants, a sentence to this effect is sufficient.

D. Language development is mentioned in three circumstances: If the child is referred specifically for a language problem, regardless of the findings; if language behavior is significantly accelerated and may be a better prognostic indicator than the current adaptive behavior; or if a previously unsuspected abnormality is detected.

E. If seizures are present, whether by history or observation, state the type and give the specific dosage schedule of medication recommended.

F. Etiology: Rarely can this be specified precisely. If antecedent factors are present, indicate that etiology may be related to them, *e.g.*, toxemia, bleeding, prematurity, illness during pregnancy. If not, indicate if the damage appears to have arisen prenatally (the usual), postnatally, or at birth.

VIII. Prognosis and Recommendations:

Indicate if average, normal, or slower than normal development is to be expected. If prognosis is guarded, state reasons. Separate intellectual from motor development when appropriate. Make specific recommendations for immediate treatment (*e.g.*, cerebral palsy clinic, seizure control, early childhood education programs, auditory training) and for the type of educational placement that might be anticipated (*e.g.*, school at regular age or with younger children, slow-learners classes in the public schools, community classes for the retarded, or rarely, institutionalization).

IX. Reexamination:

A. Thank you sentence: "We appreciate the opportunity of seeing John and would like to be kept informed of his progress."

B. State the specific time for reexamination, and whether by you or by other agencies at school age to determine educational placement. Alternatively, state no further examination is indicated unless special problems arise.

X. Indicate for your secretary what diagnoses should be entered on the patient's file card.

Illustrative Case Report (based on data entered in sample forms)

Joseph Doctor, M.D.	Re: John Doe
High Street	Birth Date: 1/1/78
Williamstown, New York 12201	CC Age: 28 weeks
	Case #: 0001

7/28/78 Developmental Consultation

John Doe is examined because the parents are puzzled about his progress in the face of a chromosomally confirmed diagnosis of trisomy 21.

John is the fifth pregnancy of this 39-year-old mother. The 15-year-old brother had a hare lip repaired with good cosmetic results. There was a miscarriage at 2 months of gestation between the births of the 12- and 10-year-olds, who are entirely normal. There is no other relevant family history. John was born 2 weeks before the expected date with a weight of 5 lb. 8 oz. There was spotting at the time of the first missed menstrual period and moderate bleeding after the onset of labor. Immediate neonatal condition was good, but there was one apneic episode on the first day of life with perhaps some subsequent cyanosis. Oxygen was given for 2 days, and he was discharged on day 6. A report from the genetics laboratory indicated the presence of trisomy 21.

John did well until 4 months of age when he had a tonic-clonic generalized seizure lasting about 30 minutes on the 3rd day of what proved to be roseola. He was discharged from the hospital after 3 days on no medication. The mother feels that after this he did not use his right arm and leg as well as before, but that he is not really handicapped significantly, and his progress has been about the same as that of her other children. There is no history of any other seizure activity, and he has had no difficulty as a result of his heart disease (a small ventricular septal defect).

John has the typical clinical appearance of trisomy 21. He makes a stable adjustment to the examination and establishes a friendly social rapport with the examiner after first sizing her up. Behavior is slightly disorganized, and exploitation is impulsive. Attention and interest tend to wander but are easily recalled to the examination situations. No seizure activity is observed.

Abnormal neuromotor patterns are present. There is mild hypotonicity of the left arm and leg and the neck, with moderate hypotonicity of the back. The right extremities show mild spasticity with increased resistance to rapid movement, but no limitation of the full range of motion. There is a moderate, alternating internal strabismus. In sitting, there is mild extension and adduction of the legs or flexion of the knees and hips, greater on the right, and moderate rounding of the back. In standing, the right leg is mildly extended and the base slightly narrow. The right arm is held slightly adducted with the elbow flexed, while the left arm has moderate abduction. There is fisting, thumb adduction, maldirected reaching, and difficulty retaining, all of which are mild on the left and of moderate degree on the right.

John shows the following behavior characteristics: *Adaptive behavior* (25 [23–27] weeks): He resecures a dropped cube, occasionally takes the cube to his mouth, has a 1-hand approach and grasp, holds 1 and grasps another of the multiple cubes, and regards the cup while holding a cube. He bangs the bell, shakes the rattle, and transfers the dangling ring, but awkwardly. *Gross motor behavior* (22 weeks): He lifts his legs high in extension, rolls to prone, holds his trunk erect in the supporting chair, is beginning to sit leaning forward on his hands, and supports a large fraction of his weight when held standing. *Fine motor behavior* (24 weeks): He grasps the cube palmarwise, more effectively on the left, and contacts a pellet. *Language behavior* (25 weeks): He turns his head to the bell-ringing, grunts and growls, and is reported to say "m-m-m." *Personal-Social behavior* (26 weeks): He discriminates strangers, vocalizes and pats at his mirror image, and bites and chews on toys. He is reported to sit propped for 30 minutes, and to take his foot to his mouth while supine.

On the Gesell Developmental and Neurologic Examination, John's general maturity level is approximately 25 weeks with some scatter; behavior is fairly well-integrated, and a low average development is indicated at the present time. He has a mild right spastic hemiplegia, superimposed on mild generalized hypotonicity, probably secondary to the grand mal convulsion at 4 months of age.

Many children with trisomy 21 show average development in early infancy and do not begin to evidence the deceleration that invariably occurs until 9–12 months of age. The functional level John will attain at maturity cannot be predicted precisely, but it is anticipated that he will have a mild degree of mental deficiency, provided no adverse circumstances supervene. He should be able to participate in special classes in the public school system. His hemiplegia should not interfere with the acquisition or exercise of motor control, but he must be observed carefully and a program of physical therapy instituted immediately if there is the slightest hint of limitation of motion. His strabismus should be evaluated by an ophthalmologist. The most important measure for maximizing his developmental potential is the prevention of subsequent convulsions, especially since his first seizure left neuromotor residua. John should be placed on daily doses of phenobarbital at 10 mg/kg and maintained on medication for at least 2 seizure-free years. A copy of the seizure control regimen we have found effective is enclosed.

The diagnosis and prognosis were discussed with the parents, who appear to have a realistic acceptance of the situation. They might benefit from contact with other parents through the local Early Childhood Education Program, and were given the address.

We appreciate the opportunity of seeing John and would like to be kept informed of his progress. Unless special problems arise, reevaluation by us is not indicated. He should have psychologic examinations at later ages in order to make plans for the best educational placement, initially in a nursery school, should the parents wish it, and later in a formal academic program.

Jane Roe, M.D.

Director, Developmental Disabilities Service

Professor of Pediatrics

cc: Division of Medical Genetics

7
Screening

Although every child needs and deserves developmental supervision, the specialist's skills should be reserved for accurate diagnosis of difficult problems. The number of children in whom abnormal development is suspected is enormous, the need for service great, and the supply of specialists limited.

Thus, there is a need for developmental screening to be carried out at a variety of levels—from parents through child-care workers, public health nurses, general practitioners, pediatricians, and other specialists who deal with children. A screening interview and examination indicate if the infant is demonstrating behavior appropriate for his age. If he is not, the particular areas involved and the extent of deviation can be determined, and a decision made about the need for referral for more detailed evaluation and the level of expertise required.

Screening for developmental disabilities should be undertaken within a total health care setting. Development cannot be treated separately from the health and welfare of the whole child. Before large scale screening programs are instituted, care must be taken to insure that facilities are available not only for a full diagnostic assessment for each child screened as abnormal or suspect, but also for the treatment or management of defects which are detected.

CRITERIA FOR AN ADEQUATE SCREENING INVENTORY

In evaluating development, one is concerned with both present and future function. The complete examination from which a screening inventory is derived must be an adequate predictor of later abnormality. First, then, it must have validity. This predictive value can be determined only by longitudinal studies, and such data derive from followup correlations between the complete early examinations and those done at later ages.

Second, since a screening inventory does not include all the behavior patterns evaluated by a complete examination, the results achieved by it must correlate with those of the full developmental evaluation. Ideally, no child called abnormal by the complete examination should be called Normal on screening (*underscreening*), and there should be a minimum of normal infants called Abnormal (*over-screening*). To determine if screening gives the same results as a complete developmental evaluation, one uses the history and observations obtained at an examination to complete the screening inventory. Then if the diagnostic classification from the inventory does not agree with that of the examination, the inventory is not likely to give satisfactory results under any other circumstances.

Third, for prediction as well as for present management, intellectual defect and motor disability must be distinguished by the inventory. Behavior must be evaluated separately in the different areas of functioning, since only adaptive and language behavior are related closely to later intellectual function. A sufficient number of items must be selected from the complete examination to permit evaluation of important developmental concepts in each area of behavior. The materials needed to accomplish the evaluation should be available readily.

Fourth, the inventory should yield reproducible results when used by different individuals observing the same examination; that is, it must be reliable. In order for this to be achieved, the behavior items in the inventory must be stated as precisely as possible, so that the examiner, observers, and the person giving the history know what is meant in each instance.

Fifth, the age intervals must be small enough so that correct diagnostic classification can be achieved even if the chronologic age of the infant lies between two inventory age levels. In the first year of life, changes occur so rapidly that items must be provided at 4-week intervals. Because they represent stages at which major integrations occur, the key ages of the developmental schedules provide the most information, but the infants may not always oblige by presenting themselves at these key ages.

Finally, supplementary information must be obtained from the parents about convulsive seizures, hearing, vision, strabismus, unilateral disabilities, the loss of previously acquired behavior, and any concerns they have about the child. Developmental quotients derived from the screening inventory are the starting points for evaluation, and the supplementary information may indicate that more detailed examination is necessary, in spite of quantitative adequacy.

In view of the limited resources to carry out even a screening process, a two-stage screening is recommended which utilizes a parent questionnaire, the Revised Parent Developmental Questionnaire (RPDQ), as the first stage. The Revised Developmental Screening Inventory (RDSI), completed by a trained child-care worker, public health nurse or primary care physician, is the second stage. The supplementary questions would accompany each stage.

THE REVISED DEVELOPMENTAL SCREENING INVENTORY

The RDSI consists of selected items from the full revised developmental schedules in each of the 5 fields of behavior. It covers the same ages from 4 weeks to 36 months. Behavior at 4, 8 and 12 weeks is dominated by reflex activity and strongly influenced by physiologic states of hunger and sleep. It is not predictive of later development. (See Chapter 1.) These ages are included only for the assessment of older abnormal infants who may be functioning at these very low levels. As already indicated, the major question for this screening inventory, as for any screening instrument, is whether it will identify all the abnormal children. Minimal overreferral of normal children is desirable.

The RDSI was developed and evaluated by comparing the diagnostic categories assigned by it with the diagnoses of intellectual potential and neuromotor status made by the complete Revised Gesell Developmental and Neurologic Examination. For a sample of 125 normal and abnormal children seen on a developmental disabilities service, the behavior recorded on the developmental schedules was transferred to the Screening Inventory. No supplementary information was included. A different physician determined maturity levels in each of the 5 areas, then the age of the child was supplied and diagnostic categories of Normal, Questionable or Abnormal were assigned for both intellectual potential and neuromotor status. The criteria used for this assignment are specified on pages 217 and 219.

Table 7–1. Comparisons of Categories Assigned by the Revised Developmental Screening Inventory and by the Revised Gesell Developmental and Neurologic Examination, Ages 16 Weeks to 36 Months

For Children

	Examination			
Screening	Normal	Questionable	Abnormal	Total
Normal	40	0	0	40
Questionable	2	34	0	36
Abnormal	0	2	47	49
Total	42	36	47	125

Underscreening:	None
Overscreening:	4/78, 5.1%
% Normal of those referred:	2/85, 2.4%

Table 7-1 indicates that all the abnormal and questionable children are detected; there are no false negatives. Two of the 42 children normal by examination are called Questionable, and 2 of the 36 questionable by examination are called Abnormal. The false-positive overreferral rate is 5%. Table 7-2 for neuromotor status and Table 7-3

Table 7–2. Comparisons of Categories Assigned by the Revised Developmental Screening Inventory and by the Revised Gesell Developmental and Neurologic Examination, Ages 16 Weeks to 36 Months

For Neuromotor Status

	Examination			
Screening	Normal	Questionable	Abnormal	Total
Normal	42	0	0	42
Questionable	3	32	0	35
Abnormal	0	2	46	48
Total	45	34	46	125

Underscreening:	None
Overscreening:	5/79, 6.3%
% Normal of those referred:	3/83, 3.6%

Table 7–3. Comparisons of Categories Assigned by the Revised Developmental Screening Inventory and by the Revised Gesell Developmental and Neurologic Examination, Ages 16 Weeks to 36 Months

For Intellectual Potential

Screening	Examination			
	Normal	Questionable	Abnormal	Total
Normal	88	2	0	90
Questionable	3	14	0	17
Abnormal	1	1	16	18
Total	92	17	16	125

Underscreening: 2/33, 6.1%
Overscreening: 5/109, 4.6%
% Normal of those referred: 4/35, 11.4%

for intellectual potential indicate that only in intellectual potential does any underscreening occur. Two children diagnosed clinically as dull normal or borderline dull, *i.e.*, questionable, are called Normal by the Screening Inventory. None of the abnormals is misclassified.

Neuromotor status and intellectual potential must be considered separately in validating the Screening Inventory, since combinations of these two attributes other than those found in the 125 children will occur. For example, a child who has questionable intellectual potential and questionable neuromotor status on examination may be detected on the basis of the neuromotor status. Another child with the same questionable intellectual potential but normal neuromotor status on examination could be missed.

Overscreening rates of normal children, for neuromotor status and intellectual potential, are 6% and 5%, respectively. Of the 85 children referred by the Inventory as Abnormal or Questionable, only 2, or 2%, are normal on examination. Of the 83 children referred on the basis of neuromotor status, 3, or 4%, are actually normal on examination. Of the 35 children referred on the basis of intellectual potential, 4, or 11%, are actually normal on examination.

These rates of under- and overreferral should be compared to the popular Denver Developmental Screening Test (DDST).[3] The percentages of abnormal and questionables by examination called Normal by the DDST, that is, the percentages of underscreening, are 9% and 38%, respectively. Of those normal on examination, 24% are overreferred. Of those referred as Abnormal or Questionable on screening,

Table 7-4. Comparison of Screening Results by Revised Developmental Screening
Inventory (RDSI) and Denver Developmental Screening Test (DDST)

Examination Category	Gesell RDSI		Frankenburg DDST	
	N	% Detected	N	% Detected
Abnormal	47	100	22	91
Questionable	36	100	34	62
Subtotal	83	100	56	73
Normal	42	95	181	76
% Abnormal of those referred	85	98	85	48
No. children screened		125		237

52% are actually called normal by the criterion tests, a DQ or IQ
score of 80 or more on the Bayley or Stanford-Binet test. Table 7-4
shows the comparison with Table 7-1.

THE REVISED PARENT DEVELOPMENTAL
QUESTIONNAIRE

Parents can be used as a primary screening source when specific
questions are asked. Again, in a time of limited resources, an effective
first-stage screening reduces large numbers to a manageable population for a second-stage screening. The Revised Parent Developmental
Questionnaire consists of selected behavior patterns from the RDSI
that parents can be expected to observe, and it covers the 5 fields of
behavior and the same age range. Groups of questions can be selected
from the total which will permit assigning developmental quotients
ranging from 60–65 to well above average for children of any of the
ages (Tables 7-5, and 7-6). Such quotients provide the basis for
assigning categories from the parents' answers and determining if a
second-stage screening is necessary. A coding system which assigns a
maturity level for each possible combination of answers and sets forth
specific criteria for assigning a diagnostic category enables a trained
clerk to make a determination of the need for referral.

The effectiveness of the parent questionnaire has been examined by
comparing the classification made on the basis of the questionnaire

Table 7–5. Age Selections for Parent Developmental Questionnaire*

Ages to Receive Questionnaire	Questionnaire "Age"	Questions Included from Ages
16–25 weeks	16 weeks	12–24 weeks
26–34 weeks	28 weeks	16–36 weeks
35–47 weeks	40 weeks	24–48 weeks
48 weeks–14 months (60 weeks)	52 weeks	32–56 weeks
(61 weeks) 14.5 months–22 months	15 months	44 weeks–21 months
22.5 months–42 months	18–36 months	18–36 months

*Questions should be selected which will permit deriving developmental quotients (DQs) ranging from less than 75 to 100 or more. This can be accomplished by incorporating questions from individual ages into six different questionnaires, as above. Table 7-5 indicates a range of developmental quotients for various maturity levels and chronologic ages.

with the results of a full Gesell Developmental and Neurologic Evaluation. In one study[3] of a group of 526 infants, the amount of underscreening, that is, calling abnormal infants Normal, was 2.6%. The rate of underscreening of infants with minor problems was 10%. Overscreening of normal infants as Questionable or Abnormal was 6%. It was determined that parents from a wide range of educational and social backgrounds could answer the questionnaire equally well. The small amount of underreferral and overreferral in combination with its effectiveness over wide social strata make this parent questionnaire an ideal first-stage screening device which can be mailed, used in the waiting rooms of physician's offices and health clinics, or carried on home visits by public health nurses.

The results with this questionnaire based on the Gesell should be compared with another popular questionnaire which evaluates parents' estimates of current behavior, the Prescreening Developmental Questionnaire (PDQ) of Frankenburg and coworkers.[4] Under- and overscreening by the PDQ is of the same order of magnitude as that found for its second-stage screening instrument, the DDST. As Table 7-7 indicates, 13% of those abnormal and 46% of those questionable on the DDST were called Normal by the PDQ, compared to 3% and 10% by the Gesell. Twenty-seven percent of the normals by DDST are overreferred, compared to 6% by the Gesell. Of those referred as Abnormal for the second-stage DDST, 77% were found to be normal, compared to the Gesell 21%.

Table 7–6. Range of Maturity Levels (columns) and Corresponding Expected Developmental Quotients (body of table) Determining the Selection of Questions from the Developmental Screening Inventory to be sent to Parents at Specified Chronologic Ages (rows).

Chronologic Age	Maturity Level																
	Weeks														Months		
	4	8	12	16	20	24	28	32	36	40	44	48	52	56	15	18	21
4w	100	(200)															
8w	50	100	150														
12w		67	100	133													
16w			75	100	125	150											
20w			60	80	100	120	140										
24w				67	83	100	117	133									
28w				57	71	86	100	114	128								
32w					63	75	88	100	113	125							
36w						67	78	89	100	111	122	133					
40w						60	70	80	90	100	110	120					
44w							64	73	82	91	100	109	118	127			
48w								67	75	83	92	100	108	117			
52w								62	69	77	84	92	100	107	125		
56w									64	71	78	86	93	100	116	139	
15m											68	74	80	86	100	120	
18m											56	62	67	72	83	100	117
21m															71	86	100

Table 7–7. Comparison of Screening Results by Gesell
Questionnaire and by Frankenburg PDQ

Examination Category	Gesell Questionnaire		Frankenburg PDQ	
	N	% Detected	N	% Detected
Abnormal	38	97	30	87
Questionable	61	90	106	54
Subtotal	99	93	136	61
Normal	427	94	1005	73
% Abnormal of those referred	117	79	356	23
Number screened	526		1141	

DEVELOPMENTAL SCREENING IN PRACTICE

In a satisfactory system of health care service, all infants would be screened and abnormalities diagnosed and treated. Under present limitations of health care services, efforts could be concentrated in "high-risk" populations—low-birth-weight infants, survivors of neonatal intensive care units, infants of teenage mothers and of those with high complication of pregnancy rates, and those from poverty areas. It is in these populations, rather than in populations where the rate of abnormality is low, that early intervention is likely to minimize more of the costs of lifetime care and loss of productivity.

It is possible to identify on the basis of prenatal and neonatal characteristics a certain number of infants within a newborn intensive care unit at very high risk for developmental disabilities. These infants should be followed closely and screened at a very early age. Otherwise, a parent questionnaire at 28 weeks of age for other infants in high-risk groups, followed by a second-stage screening for those categorized as Abnormal or Questionable, will identify almost all infants with organic disease of the central nervous system who will need definitive diagnosis and early intervention of some kind: control of seizures; treatment of cerebral palsy with a program of supervised passive exercises if not the full range of services of a Cerebral Palsy Treatment Center; hearing aids and auditory training programs; support and guidance for parents of mentally retarded and blind infants; tagging for followup of those infants at risk for later school failure; and the initiation of preschool programs and early institution of remedial school programs where warranted.

Developmental problems can surface at any age. However, the normal infant develops normally unless some noxious event, either organic or sociocultural, occurs. It is unlikely that many cases of meningitis, major seizures, brain tumors or significant head trauma will be missed. Those normal infants who later fail in school because they come from an impoverished and nonacademic environment are detectable between 2 and 3 years of age. They can be identified early from a variety of demographic data, most of which can be obtained from birth certificates.

However, it is precisely in the low sociocultural group, which provides the largest number who will fail in school, where the return rate of a mailed questionnaire is lowest. Inner-city and very rural families are the ones who also have difficulties in keeping appointments. They usually have little money or other resources, have no telephones, and are apt to move frequently. A mailed parental questionnaire is not sufficient for reaching this population, and a more direct home-visiting program is necessary. Limited resources should be concentrated in these areas of greatest need and yield, with the use of instruments that generate the fewest possible false negatives and false positives.

THE SUPPLEMENTARY QUESTIONS

A cover letter which explains the purpose of the questionnaire to the parents and gives instructions for completing it also contains the questions which must supplement the behavior patterns. The answers to these questions should be obtained by the individual using the Screening Inventory as well.

- Does (s)he turn to look at you when you talk in a normal voice?
- Do you think (s)he hears?
- Has (s)he ever had any convulsions or fits?
- Does (s)he ever stare off into space and keep right on staring if you put your hand in front of his/her eyes and *hold* it there?
- Does (s)he ever start to cry for no apparent reason and keep right on crying no matter what you do to try to comfort him/her?
- Does (s)he have a lazy eye or squint?
- Some children look as though their eyes are crossing because of the wide space between them. The way to tell the differ-

ence between these children and those whose eyes really cross is to see where the reflections of a light, or a window, appear in the colored part of the eyes.

- Are these reflections in the same place in both eyes, no matter in what direction the child is looking, as in this picture?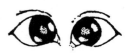
- Is there anything about your child that worries you? Explain. If yes, how old was (s)he when you began to worry?
- Has (s)he ever lost behavior once achieved?
- Does (s)he use both hands equally well? Both feet?
  Is your child taking any medication?
      What is it?
      What is the dose per day?
- What age child do you think your child is acting like?
      How his/her mind works?
      Controlling his/her body and hands?
      Making sounds or talking?
      Understanding what you say?

THE INVENTORY

THE REVISED DEVELOPMENTAL SCREENING INVENTORY—4 WEEKS TO 36 MONTHS

THE OBJECTIVE OF DEVELOPMENTAL SCREENING IS TO DETERMINE IF A CHILD IS FUNCTIONING AT AGE LEVEL OR IF THERE IS SOME ABNORMALITY INDICATING THAT MORE DETAILED EXAMINATION IS REQUIRED. This inventory is a screening procedure, and a definitive diagnosis should not be made on the basis of its use. Some children identified as abnormal will require prompt referral to a consultant or a center for a complete diagnostic evaluation. Other children will require serial observations to determine if such referral is necessary.

FIRST: READ THE INSTRUCTIONS ON PAGES 217 THROUGH 223, AS WELL AS THE ENTIRE INVENTORY, BEFORE ATTEMPTING TO USE IT.

Enter the child's name and other identifying information on page 210 of the Inventory. Age in weeks, through 56 weeks, should be calculated from a clendar. Half *months* may be used from 13.5 months on. When indicated, calculate a CORRECTED BIRTH DATE by ADDING the days of PREMATURITY to the actual birth date. Use the Corrected Birth Date for determining CORRECTED CHRON-OLOGIC AGE for each evaluation done.

ASK parents questions appropriate to the child's *age* and *function;* RECORD their answers in the HISTORY (H) column. When you start your interview TELL THE PARENTS SOME QUESTIONS ASKED WILL BE ABOVE THE CHILD'S LEVEL OF ABILITIES.

RECORD your observations in the OBSERVATION (O) column. RECORD responses as +(Present), −(Absent), X(unknown), ±(if behavior is between 2 age levels, or is seen only occasionally and is not the dominant pattern).

On page 218 ASSIGN AGE MATURITY LEVELS in each of the 5 areas of behavior, in weeks or months, based on your clinical judgment of the age levels your recorded history and observations describe best. See page 217 for further elaboration of this point.

Assign a DIAGNOSTIC CATEGORY in each area on the basis of your age levels. DO NOT EXPECT TO MAKE A PRECISE DIAG-NOSIS, but assign the child to one of three categories: A (definitely ABNORMAL); Q (borderline or QUESTIONABLY abnormal); N (NORMAL or advanced). See page 219 for additional guidance on this point.

DO NOT BE ALARMED BY THE LARGE NUMBER OF QUESTIONS. They cover the age range from 1 to 36 months, and any *one* child usually can be evaluated by 2 or 3 consecutive age levels in any given area of behavior.

Case #: _____

Last Name _____

First Name _____

Birth Date: _____

Birth Weight: _____

E.D.C.: _____

Days Prematurity Assigned: _____

Corrected Birth Date: _____

	H	O	KEY AGE: 4 Weeks or less	H	O	8 Weeks
ADAPTIVE	▓		Regard toy only when brought in front of eyes			Follow dangled *ring* past midline
			Follow dangled toy only to mid-line, not past it			Follow dangled *ring* vertically, both up and down
			Facial expression or stopping activity in response to sound			
GROSS MOTOR			Asymmetric tonic-neck-reflex postures predominate			Head bob erect if held sitting
			Head sag forward if held sitting			No head droop, suspended prone
			Clear nose from bed, prone			Lift head to 45° recurrently, prone (on abdomen)
FINE MOTOR			Both hands held tightly fisted			Hold dangling ring put in hand briefly
		▓	Clench hand as toy touched to it			
LANGUAGE			Impassive face			Alert expression
			Vague indirect regard	▓		Direct definite regard
					▓	Coo (oooo, aaah)
PERSONAL-SOCIAL			Regard examiner's face and decrease activity			Eyes follow moving person around
			Indefinite stare at surroundings			Smile and talk back just if you nod your head and talk

	12 Weeks	16 Weeks (KEY AGE)	20 Weeks
ADAPTIVE	Prompt regard of toy dangled in midline at chest level	Wave arms, move body at sight of dangled toy, on back	Bring both hands towards dangled toy, on back
	Regard cup-sized toy on table, supported sitting	Look at toy in hand, on back	Grasp toy only if held near palm (about 1 inch away)
	Glance at toy put into hand	Take toy to mouth, on back	Look after toy dropped in sight
		Wave arms at sight of cube on table, supported sitting	Bring both hands toward cube
GROSS MOTOR	Head bob forward, held sitting	Head steady, set forward, sitting	Lift legs high, see toes, on back
	Symmetric postures head, body predominate	*Hold* head 90°, look directly ahead, prone (on abdomen)	No head lag, held by hands and pulled to sitting
	Hold head up 45° sustainedly, prone	Roll from abdomen to back	Push whole chest off bed, prone, both elbows straight
FINE MOTOR	Hold hands open, or close loosely	Curl fingers actively around toy touched to hand	Retain placed cube momentarily, lifting it off tabletop
	Scratch, finger, clutch at clothes	Scratch on tabletop, or on bed, prone	
LANGUAGE	Chuckle	Laugh out loud	Grunt and growl (deep sounds) not with bowel movement
		Squeal (high-pitched sounds)	
PERSONAL-SOCIAL	Recognize bottle on sight	Initiate smile just when people come and stand beside him	Lick and mouth toy
	Hold up and look at own hand	Pat bottle with both hands	Know difference between family and strangers
		Smile and talk to self, if *close* to large mirror	

READ INSTRUCTIONS

H = History; O = Observation

	H	O	24 Weeks	H	O	KEY AGE: 28 Weeks	H	O	32 Weeks
ADAPTIVE			Reach for and secure toy with both hands, supine and sitting			Reach and pick up cube with 1 hand only			Pick up cube in each hand and hold both more than 1 minute
			Reach for toy dropped in reach, supine (on back)			Pick up cube in each hand			Hit cube in hand at cube on table
			Put cube in mouth, held sitting			Transfer toy easily hand to hand			Take cube out of cup
			Resecure cube from table			Bang toy up and down, held in sitting			
GROSS MOTOR			Roll to abdomen, get both arms out from under chest			Sit erect 1 minute on *hard* surface			Sit 10 + minutes steady on *hard* surface
			Sit well leaning on hands if placed on *hard* surface			Stand hands held shoulder height, elbows fully extended			Stand at furniture and not lean against it, if put there
			Support full weight and bounce, held around chest			Get up on hands and knees			
FINE MOTOR			Pick up cube and hold in center of palm with all fingers			Pick up cube, hold to radial palm with 2nd and 3rd fingers			Pick up pellet, using all fingers and thumb
			Put whole hand on pellet or string, rake it			Try to pick up pellet, raking with thumb, 2nd, 3rd fingers			
LANGUAGE			Turn head to sound			Make single consonant sounds: da, ba, ga, a-da			Say da-da, ba-ba without meaning
						Imitate cough, tongue-click, etc.			Respond to No-No, tone of voice
PERSONAL-SOCIAL			Grasp feet, lying on back			Feet to mouth, lying on back			Feed self cracker, do good job
			Pat image when put *close* to large mirror			Bite and chew, not just lick, toys			Take *milk*, not just water and juice, from cup or glass

	H	O	36 Weeks	H	O	KEY AGE: 40 Weeks	H	O	44 Weeks
ADAPTIVE			Hold bottle and try to or pick up pellet at same time			Poke at pellet inside bottle			Put cube inside cup but not let go of it
			Poke index finger at things		▓	Bang 2 cubes together in air, pat-a-cake fashion			Uncover cube you have placed under a piece of paper
						Use string to secure attached ring, see connection			
GROSS MOTOR			Sit erect, steady indefinitely			Hold furniture with both hands and walk around it			Hold furniture with 1 hand and walk around it
			Creep (crawl) on hands and knees			Let self down from furniture with control			Walk if both hands held shoulder height for balance only
			Pull self to full standing position						
FINE MOTOR			Pick up cube, *ends* of fingers			Pluck pellet up with *tips* of thumb and index finger, arm and hand resting on table			Put cube down, take hand off
			Pick up pellet, thumb and sides of index finger						
LANGUAGE			Say any 1 "word"			Say any 2 "words"			Say any 3 "words"
			"Sing along" with music			Play nursery game just if asked			Follow simple *verbal* commands
PERSONAL-SOCIAL			Hold own bottle, pick up if dropped and finish it			Extend toy to you, but not let go of it			Release toy into your hand, if you hold your hand out for it
			Imitate 2 nursery games, if you start them first			Push arm through sleeve once it is started in			Lift foot for shoe or diaper

H = History O = Observations   READ INSTRUCTIONS

	H	O	48 Weeks	H	O	KEY AGE: 52 Weeks	H	O	56 Weeks
ADAPTIVE			Try piling 1 cube on 2nd, but it falls off			Dangle toy by string, deliberate			Put all of 9–10 cubes into cup
			Put 2 cubes into cup in sequence			Drop pellet into bottle			Try to get toy with stick, demonstration
			Try to put pellet into bottle, release without success			Imitate back-and-forth scribble made with crayon			Stroke crayon in air after vertical stroke drawn
GROSS MOTOR			Walk straight forward with 1 hand held			Pick up toy from floor without holding on for support			No longer creep or crawl
			Take a few steps from object to object			Get up in middle of floor and take several steps alone			Climb into adult chair
FINE MOTOR			Pluck pellet easily with *tips* of thumb and index finger, not resting arm or hand on table			Help turn pages of a book			Pile 1 cube on 2nd (Tower 2)
						Throw ball with good cast			
LANGUAGE			Say 4 "words"			Say 6 "words"			Say 8 "words"
			Look at *object* when asked: ball, shoe, light, TV, etc.			Pat at pictures in book			Get object from another room on request
PERSONAL-SOCIAL			Play ball with you			Indicate wants by pointing			— — — —
						Hug or love doll, stuffed toy			

		15 Months			KEY AGE: 18 Months			21 Months
H	**O**		**H**	**O**		**H**	**O**	
ADAPTIVE		Put all of 9–10 cubes into cup			Imitate *pushing* train of cubes that has been made			Align 3 cubes for train
		Dump pellet from bottle if shown			Dump pellet from bottle, on request			Try to get toy with stick, without demonstration
		Get toy with stick, after demonstration			Imitate stroke on paper after vertical stroke drawn			
		Scribble spontaneously when given crayon						
GROSS MOTOR		Stack 3 cubes (Tower 3)			Walk down stairs, 1 hand held			Run well
					Walk into or step on large ball when shown how to kick it			Walk up or down stairs, holding rail
FINE MOTOR		Rarely fall when walking			Stack 4 cubes (Tower 4)			Stack 6 cubes (Tower 6)
		Run stiff-legged			Turn book pages 2–3 at once			
		Climb on chair to reach things						
LANGUAGE		Vocabulary of 10–19 words			Combine 2 ideas (Daddy bye, car go)			Vocabulary of 30–50 words
		Point to 1 body part on request			Point to picture in book			Name 1 picture in book
					Point to 4 body parts on request			Identify 4 test objects
					Follow 2 directional commands with ball, block			Follow 4 directional commands with ball or block
PERSONAL-SOCIAL		Leave dish on tray when fed			Hand empty dish when done			Eat with fork
		Use spoon, spill good bit			Use regular cup or glass, put down when finished			Pretend to feed, dress doll
		Pull persons to show them things			Imitate mopping, dusting, etc.			Unzip own zippers

READ INSTRUCTIONS

H = History O = Observation

	H	O	KEY AGE: 24 Months	H	O	30 Months	H	O	KEY AGE: 36 Months
ADAPTIVE			Align all 4 cubes for train			Add chimney to train			Imitate bridge
			Imitate vertical stroke			Imitate horizontal stroke			Copy circle
			Get toy with stick on request			Imitate circle			Imitate cross
						Repeat 2 digits, 1 of 3 trials			Repeat 3 digits, 1 of 3 trials
GROSS MOTOR			Jump, both feet off floor			Alternate feet going up stairs			Alternate feet going down stairs
			Kick ball on request			Stand on 1 foot momentarily			Do broad jump, both feet
FINE MOTOR			Stack 7 cubes (Tower 7)			Stack 9 cubes (Tower 9)			Stack 10 cubes (Tower 10)
			Thread shoelace through safety pin hole			Turn pages in book singly			Hold crayon adult fashion
									Try to cut with scissors
LANGUAGE			Use "I" or "you"			Give action in picture			Give use of 2 test objects
		▨	Say 3–4 word sentences		▨	Name all 7 body parts			Give full name
			Identify action in picture			Indicate use of key or penny			Identify 2 colors
			Point to all 7 body parts			Follow 2 prepositional commands with ball or block			Follow 3 prepositional commands with ball or block
PERSONAL-SOCIAL			Feed self, spill little			Pour well from glass to glass			Toilet trained, dry at night
			Push stroller, etc., steer well			Find armholes in coat correctly			Understand taking turns
			Allowed to carry breakables			Name mirror image			Dress self with supervision

H = History   O = Observation   READ INSTRUCTIONS

Instructions

TOWER: 15–36 Months is *both* ADAPTIVE *and* FINE MOTOR. Must be 1-inch cubes.
   Fine Motor: Number built without examiner's holding to help.
   Adaptive: Examiner may hold if child brings successive cubes to tower but has motor disability stopping precise release.

TAKE TOWER INTO ACCOUNT IN
ASSIGNING ADAPTIVE AGE LEVEL

COPY: Reproduce from model
IMITATE: After demonstration. Ask to copy, name, etc., before imitating, pointing.

TRAIN: ■■■■ Demonstrate out of reach; say, "One car, another car, another, and the chimney for the smoke," push train and say, "choo-choo."
   Imitating pushing: Child slides cube along, or moves hand says, "choo."

BRIDGE: ■■■
   Copy: Point to model; say, "Here is downstairs, the door, upstairs."
   Imitate: Say, "One like this, one like this, one like this," then point as for *copy.*
TEST OBJECTS: Pencil, key, penny, examiner's shoe, ball.
DIGITS: Child repeats *only* after examiner says entire set of 2 or 3: 4–2, 6–3, 5–8, 6–4–1, 3–5–2, 8–3–7
COMMANDS: Request only; no pointing
   Directions: Put on table, on chair, give to mother, to me.
   Prepositions: On, under, in back of (behind), in front of, beside.

Blocks are provided on page 218 for recording the age levels at which the child is functioning, and the diagnoses. In each of the 5 areas of behavior assign maturity age levels in weeks or months. The maturity level is assigned by determining how well a child's behavior fits one age level constellation rather than another. The maturity level is that point at which the aggregate of *plus* signs changes to an aggregate of *minus* signs. For example, if a 40-week old has all + signs at 40 weeks, 1 + at 44 weeks and 1 + at 48 weeks, an age level of 42 weeks would be assigned as approximating most closely the child's maturity. Thus, interpolation between adjacent levels is done, since a 40-week-old infant adds behavior gradually in achieving a 44-week level of function. When wide scatter and gaps are present within one area,

Record the Results of Each Evaluation in the Spaces Below:

Date							
Age							
ADAPTIVE BEHAVIOR	Maturity Level Assigned / DQ						
	Diagnostic Category						
GROSS MOTOR BEHAVIOR	Maturity Level Assigned / DQ						
	Diagnostic Category						
FINE MOTOR BEHAVIOR	Maturity Level Assigned / DQ						
	Diagnostic Category						
LANGUAGE BEHAVIOR	Maturity Level Assigned / DQ						
	Diagnostic Category						
PERSONAL-SOCIAL BEHAVIOR	Maturity Level Assigned / DQ						
	Diagnostic Category						
FINAL DIAGNOSTIC CATEGORY							

READ INSTRUCTIONS

assign a range and average it to determine the DQ (see below). DO NOT FORGET TO TAKE THE PARENTS' HISTORY INTO ACCOUNT. This is particularly important for assessing language behavior, which may not be exhibited during the examination. We have found parents' reports to be very accurate when clear-cut, specific questions are asked.

Calculate a Developmental Quotient (DQ) for each area.

$$\frac{\text{Maturity age level}}{\text{Chronologic age}} \times 100 = DQ$$

ASSIGN Diagnostic Categories to each area:

A (Abnormal) if DQ is 75 or less.
Q (Questionable) if DQ is between 76 and 85.
N (Normal) if DQ is 86 or more.

ASSIGN A FINAL DIAGNOSTIC CATEGORY:

A (Abnormal) if *either* ADAPTIVE *or* GROSS MOTOR DQ are 75 or less.
Q (Questionable) if ADAPTIVE or GROSS MOTOR DQs are 76–85, or FINE MOTOR *only* is 75 or less.
N (Normal) if the above areas are 86 or more.

Delayed language is not significant if the ADAPTIVE behavior is normal and you are sure the child HEARS and UNDERSTANDS what is heard.

GENERAL INSTRUCTIONS: READ THE ENTIRE INVENTORY BEFORE ATTEMPTING TO USE IT.

Development proceeds in an orderly, predictable manner with the same variability in behavior for normal children found in all biologic measurements. By asking some questions of parents, observing the child's behavior and recording the information systematically, an estimate of the level of function in various areas of behavior can be made which correlates with the maturity age assigned on the basis of a complete Revised Gesell Developmental and Neurologic Examination, from which the items are adapted.

This screening inventory will be of value for serial observations in well-baby supervision, and for determining if patients with suspected developmental problems need additional referral for diagnostic evaluation.

We have tried to phrase the items as clearly as possible. Specific explanations for some are listed on a following page. It will help to understand them if you *look at the adjacent age levels*, *e.g.*, *lift* as opposed to *hold* at 8 and 12 weeks in Gross Motor Behavior. Offer the parents both alternatives. ASK THE ITEMS AS THEY ARE STATED—DO NOT PARAPHRASE. For behavior which depends on your own observations only, the history column is blocked out. Usually you will observe the Adaptive and Motor behavior patterns.

START by asking questions appropriate to the chronologic age of the child, unless your preliminary information or observation indicates obvious delay. If answers are negative, drop to a lower age level and work back up. Continue to ask questions until no more positive answers are obtained. It is best to COVER ONE AREA OF BEHAVIOR AT A TIME rather than one age level at a time. Don't ask a question if the parents have already provided the answer in response to one asked previously.

If an infant is seen frequently there may be some overlap in behavior. Confusion may be avoided by recording in different colors. Failure to progress normally will be obvious if significant overlap between visits is present.

CONDUCT OF THE EXAMINATION

Examination Materials

In the full examination, test objects are very specific but they can be approximated. The following items can be purchased in most supermarkets or "Woolworths:"

- 4-inch round embroidery hoop; string 10 inches long, $^3/_{32}$ inches thick
- Aluminum cup, 3.75 inches in diameter, 12-ounce capacity
- Clear plastic bottle 2 inches high, 1-inch diameter (most pharmacies)
- Cinnamon "red hots;" the pellets, which come on paper strips as shoe buttons, liberty streamers, can be found
- Child's picture book
- Large crayon and paper
- 10 1-inch wooden cubes*. The surface should not be embossed with designs. Usual available size is 1¼ inches

---

*1-inch wooden cubes may be purchased from Ideal School Supply, 11000 Lavergne Ave., Oak Lawn, IL 60453, or from Milton Bradley, Springfield, MA 01101.

- Dowel stick—8 inches long, ⅜ inches in diameter is a good size; pipe cleaner "dog" makes a good small toy
- 1-inch safety pin and stiff shoelace which just fits through eye of pin

Even these objects are not essential. On the hospital wards, tongue blades, a stethoscope, or a small flashlight can be used early. Except for tower and other building, small medicine cups, pop-apart beads or other small toys infants have can substitute for the cubes. If you are very quick at inhibiting eating, a piece of paper rolled into a *small* ball is a pellet. Tape used to tie toys across the cribs is rather large, but it can substitute for the string. A large notebook or file folder can serve as a table if no tray is handy. The mother, a nurse or an attendant can support the young infant in sitting.

General Comments on Conducting the Examination

The infant must cooperate if information useful in assessing behavior is to be obtained, and the degree of cooperation often is related directly to the manner of the examiner. If you talk to the child before and during the examination in a friendly manner and do not push performance, good rapport usually is established. If it does not follow immediately upon some painful procedure, the examination often is more successful, but even in such situations presenting the toys usually will secure cooperation. OFFER SOME TOY OTHER THAN A TEST OBJECT BEFORE HANDLING THE CHILD. WHEN HE TAKES IT HE USUALLY HAS ACCEPTED YOU AND WILL PARTICIPATE IN THE EXAMINATION.

MOST BEHAVIOR IN INFANCY IS SEEN DURING SPON-TANEOUS PLAY AND NOT ELICITED ON COMMAND (*e.g.*, present one cube, then the second, add the third, the rest of the cubes, then the cup and observe the behavior). ALWAYS GIVE A CHILD AN OPPORTUNITY FOR SHOWING THE MOST AD-VANCED BEHAVIOR FIRST: spontaneous behavior; grasp before placing in hand; request before demonstration; copying before imitat-ing; naming before pointing.

REMOVE OBJECT(S) at the end of each situation or group of related situations before presenting the next one, but HAVE THE NEXT OBJECT READY before trying to take away the one in hand. IF THERE IS STRONG OBJECTION, PRESENT THE NEXT ONE BEFORE TRYING FURTHER. This procedure usually works. DO NOT USE FORCE.

Talk to the infant, or better, describe what is happening while you are doing the examination.

Presentation of the Examination Materials

Screening is not very productive prior to 16 weeks. 4–12 weeks are included for determining if an older infant has significant retardation. At 16, 20 and 24 weeks, Adaptive and Fine Motor behavior are elicited in both the supine and sitting positions. Before independent sitting is achieved, support must be provided to leave the infant's hands free for manipulation. At 28 weeks and beyond, the *normal* infant need not be placed on his back. *With this exception,* ALL *INFANTS* SHOULD BE EVALUATED WHILE SUPINE, SITTING, PRONE, AND STANDING. Start with the supine position at 16 and 20 weeks, unless the mother says the infant resents this. Older infants lying in hospital cribs should be offered a toy before being changed to sitting.

Supine: Start with the object in the midline at the infant's feet and bring it up toward eye level. Hold it about 10–12 inches from the infant for visual responses and within reach if he is mature enough to grasp.

Sitting: Tap the object at the far edge of the table in the midline with clear vertical motions of the arm. When the infant has fixated upon it, slide it *within reach* with a smooth horizontal motion; do not jerk your arm up and down. When presenting ring-string, put the string down within the infant's reach, tap the *ring* for attention, then put the ring down out of reach.

Ambulatory: For children old enough to sit at a small table, simply place the materials within reach in front of them.

SPECIFIC BEHAVIOR PATTERNS

Supine (on back):

4 Weeks: *Asymmetrical* tonic-neck-reflex (TNR). Head to side, arm and leg extended on same side; opposite arm and leg flexed, hand at occiput. The fencing position.

20 Weeks: Gets legs high enough in extension to see toes, but cannot grasp them.

Head Control in Sitting (needs full trunk support):

16 Weeks: Head not yet held in line with body; does not bob forward unless it turns to side or whole body moves.

Sitting:

24 + weeks: must be on *hard* surface, not bed.

36 Weeks: sits well enough so mother will leave room.

Grasp:

Reach out and pick up in one motion; differs from approach with eventual prehension. Progresses from ulnar (pinkie) side of hand to radial digits.

Cube Grasp:

28 Weeks: Cube still in palm, but at radial side.

36 weeks: Space between cube and palm.

Pellet Grasp:

32 Weeks: 4th and 5th fingers flex during grasp.

36 Weeks: 4th and 5th fingers suppressed completely.

48 Weeks: Adult grasp, coming down from above.

Miscellaneous:

44 Weeks: Crude release is controlled removal of hand from object, not just dropping.

44 Weeks–15 Months: All 10 cubes and cup on table for cubes and cup behavior.

48 + Weeks: Toy out of child's reach, within stick's.

24 Months: Tape up all but nonworking end of safety pin.

Language:

24 Weeks: Audubon Bird Call excellent for high-pitched soft sounds. Test in supine position before 28 weeks. Continue testing until there is specific evidence of receptive or expressive language.

36 + Weeks: "Word" is sound used consistently for person, object, group of objects. Ask for common first ones besides mama, dada: hi, bye, no, see, huh, oh-oh.

36 + Weeks: Nursery game—wave bye-bye, play pat-a-cake, peek-a-boo, so big, etc.

18 Months: "What's that," "All gone," "Big boy," essentially single words, not two separate ideas.

Personal-Social:

24 Months: "Steer well" means backs out of corners also.

THE QUESTIONNAIRE

Group 1—(ADAPTIVE)

	YES	NO
DOES YOUR CHILD		
A. Follow a toy you dangle in front of his eyes to the midline but not past it?	—	—
(4w) Change his facial expression in response to a sound near his ears?	—	—
B. Follow the toy you dangle in front of her eyes past the midline?	—	—
(8w)		
C. Look at a cup-sized toy on the table when you support him in a sitting position?	—	—
(12w) Glance at a toy briefly when it is put in his hand?	—	—
D. Wave her arms and move her body at the sight of a toy dangled in front of her when she is lying on her back or when you support her in a sitting position?	—	—
Look directly at a toy which you have put in her hand so you are sure she is looking at it?	—	—
(16w) Take a toy which you have put in her hand to her mouth when she is lying on her back? ..	—	—
E. Turn his head to look for a toy that he drops when he is on his back?	—	—
Bring both his hands directly toward a toy in front of him when he is on his back, or when (20w) you support him in a sitting position?	—	—
F. Usually reach for and pick up a toy in front of her with both hands at once?	—	—
Reach for a toy she has dropped when she is lying on her back if it is within her sight?	—	—
(24w) Put a toy she has picked up into her mouth when you support her in a sitting position? ...	—	—

G. Usually reach for and pick up a toy in front of him with only one hand? .... — |
   Put a toy back and forth directly from one hand to the other? .... — |
   (28w) Bang a toy up and down on a table or his lap when you support him in a sitting position? . — |

H. Hit a toy in her hand against one on the table? .... — |
   Pick up one small toy (about 1 inch in size) in each hand and hold these 2 toys she has
   (32w) picked up herself for more than a minute? .... — |

I. Hold a small toy (about 1 inch in size) in one hand and at the same time try to or pick up
   a smaller object such as a pea-sized crumb or Cheerio with the other? .... — |
   (36w) Poke at things or into holes with a single finger? .... — |

J. Poke at a pea-sized crumb (Cheerio) inside a clear bottle? .... — |
   (40w) Bang 2 small toys together in the air, pat-a-cake fashion? .... — |

K. If you drop a small toy (about 1 inch in size) inside a cup or box first, put it back in but
   not let go of it? .... — |
   Definitely look for a small toy he watches you hide under a piece of paper or a cloth, not
   (44w) just pull the paper off and play with it? .... — |

L. Put 2 small toys into a cup or a box one after the other? .... — |
   (48w) Try to put a pea-sized crumb into a bottle (pill bottle size), but not succeed? .... — |

M. Succeed in dropping a pea-sized crumb (Cheerio) into a bottle (2-inch pill bottle)? .... — |
   (52w) Imitate a back-and-forth scribble you have made with a crayon? .... — |

225

DOES YOUR CHILD... YES NO

N. Put all but one of 9 or 10 small toys into a cup or box? .... —— ——

Try to drag in a small toy placed slightly out of reach with a pencil, after you have shown

(56w) her how? .... —— ——

O. Scribble back and forth when you just hand him a crayon or pencil or pencil and ask him to write? .. —— ——

Succeed in getting a small toy placed slightly out of reach with a pencil, after you have

(15m) shown him how? .... —— ——

P. Watch a pea-sized crumb (Cheerio) fall out of a bottle when she turns it upside down to

get it out, without your showing her how? (It does not just fall out by accident when

she shakes the bottle.) .... —— ——

Make a definite stroke, even if it is not vertical in direction, if you make a vertical stroke

(18m) down the side of a piece of paper and ask her to imitate it? ...... —— ——

Q. If you line up 4 blocks to make a train, saying, "Here's one car, another and another,"

does he clearly imitate your train by aligning 3 of the blocks? .... —— ——

Try to get a toy placed slightly out of reach with a pencil just if you ask him to, without

(21m) your showing him first? .... —— ——

R. If you line up 4 blocks to make a train, saying, "Here's one car, another and another,"

does she clearly imitate your train by aligning all 4 blocks? ■■■■ ...... —— ——

Succeed in getting a toy placed slightly out of reach with a pencil if you ask her to, without

(24m) your showing her first? .... —— ——

S. If you line up 4 blocks to make a train and put a 5th block on top of one of the end blocks, saying, "And here's the chimney for the smoke," does he align the blocks in imitation and then add the chimney?

(You may say, "Now put the chimney on," without pointing, if he only aligns the blocks.)

(30m) Make a definite circle or series of circles, if you make a circle on a piece of paper and ask him to imitate it? .... —— ——

T. Imitate the bridge if you make one in front of her, leave it standing, and ask her to make

one just like it with some more blocks? .... —— ——

(36m) Make a cross, if you draw one first and ask her to imitate it? .... —— ——

Group 2—(GROSS MOTOR)

DOES YOUR CHILD .... **YES NO**

  A. Keep his head turned to the side most of the time? .... —— ——

(4w) Lift his head enough to clear his nose from the bed, when he is lying on his abdomen? ...... —— ——

  B. When you support her in a sitting position, hold her head straight up for a moment? .... —— ——

(8w) Lift her head up so her chin is 3—4 inches from the bed, when she is lying on her abdomen? .. —— ——

227

Group 2—(GROSS MOTOR, *continued*)

DOES YOUR CHILD .... YES NO

C. Keep his head in the midline or move it freely from side to side most of the time, on his back?. . — —
     When he is lying on his abdomen, *hold* his head up for more than 1 minute so his chin is 3–4
(12w) inches from the bed? .... — —

D. Hold her head steady when you support her in a sitting position? .... — —
     Hold her head straight up for more than one minute and look directly ahead, when she is lying
(16w) on her abdomen? .... — —

E. Keep his head in line with his body when you pull him to sitting by holding his hands? .... — —
     Straighten both elbows out and push his whole chest off the bed, when he is lying on his
(20w) abdomen? .... — —

F. Roll from her back to her abdomen and get both arms out from under herself? .... — —
     Sit with a straight back if you prop her leaning on her hands on a *hard* surface? .... — —
     Support most of her weight and bounce while standing if you hold her around the chest under
(24w) her arms? .... — —

G. Sit up straight for about 1 minute without leaning on his hands for support, when you place
     him on a *hard surface* such as the floor or a table? .... — —
     Stand and support his whole weight if you hold his hands at *shoulder height* and his elbows
     straight, only to balance him? .... — —
(28w) Get up on his hands and knees? .... — —

H.   Sit up straight for more than 10 minutes without leaning on her hands for support, when you place her on a *hard surface* such as the floor? .... ——

(32w)   Stand holding on to furniture or her crib rail without leaning her chest against it for support, if you put her there? .... ——

I.   Sit up straight and steady indefinitely, without leaning on his hands, so you can put him on the floor and go away and leave him? .... ——

  Move forward while up on his hands and knees? .... ——

(36w)   Pull himself up to a full standing position on the furniture or his crib rail? .... ——

J.   Hold furniture or her crib rail with both hands and walk along it? .... ——

(40w)   Let herself down from a standing position at the furniture or the crib rail with control? .... ——

K.   Walk well if you hold both of his hands to balance him, but without helping him support his weight? .... ——

(44w)   Hold furniture or the crib rail with one hand only and walk along it? .... ——

L.   Walk straight forward with one hand held just for balance? .... ——

(48w)   Take a few steps from object to object? .... ——

M.   Pick up a toy from the floor without holding on to any object for support? .... ——

(52w)   Get up in the middle of the floor and take several steps alone, without having to pull himself up on something first? .... ——

Group 2—(CROSS MOTOR, *continued*)

	YES	NO
DOES YOUR CHILD		
N. No longer go about on her hands and knees but walk *alone* all the time, without pulling up first?	—	—
(56w) Climb into a couch or an adult chair?	—	—
O. Fall very little when walking?	—	—
(15m) Climb on a chair or a stool in order to reach things?	—	—
P. *Walk* down stairs if you hold 1 hand?	—	—
(18m) Walk into or step on a large ball, after you have shown her how to kick it?	—	—
Q. Run well and stop himself, without having to run into a wall or piece of furniture?	—	—
(21m) *Walk* up or down stairs by himself if he holds on to the railing or the wall? . . .	—	—
R. Jump and get both feet off the floor at the same time?	—	—
(24m) Kick a ball with good leg motion and without holding on, just if you ask her to? . .	—	—
S. Alternate his feet, walking up stairs the way an adult does, 1 foot to each step? . . .	—	—
(30m) Stand balanced on 1 foot for a moment without holding on?	—	—
T. Alternate her feet going down stairs the way an adult does, 1 foot to each step? . . .	—	—
(36m) Do a broad jump, covering distance and jumping with both feet at the same time? . .	—	—

Group 3—(FINE MOTOR BEHAVIOR)

DOES YOUR CHILD ....

	YES	NO

A. Hold both hands tightly fisted when he is awake? .... ___ ___
(4w)

B. Hold a very light-weight toy you put in her hand for more than a minute? .... ___ ___
(8w)

C. Holds his hands open or loosely closed instead of tightly fisted?
Scratch and clutch at his clothes? .... ___ ___
(12w)

D. Scratch on a tabletop when held in sitting position, or on a bed when on her abdomen? .... ___ ___
(16w)

E. Pick up a small toy (about 1 inch in size) and hold it in the center of her palm with all of her
fingers? .... ___ ___
Succeed in touching a pea-sized crumb (Cheerio) with her whole hand (usually her whole arm
moves while she tries to do this)? .... ___ ___
(24w)

F. Try to pick up a pea-sized crumb (Cheerio) by using his thumb and all his fingers, without
success? .... ___ ___
(28w)

G. Pick up a pea-sized crumb (Cheerio) by curling all her fingers and bringing her thumb against
them? .... ___ ___
(32w)

231

Group 3—(FINE MOTOR BEHAVIOR, *continued*)

	YES	NO
DOES YOUR CHILD		
H. Pick up a small toy (about 1 inch in size) with the ends of his fingers?	—	—
(36w) Pick up a pea-sized crumb (Cheerio) by bringing the thumb and the side of *1* finger (usually the 1st) together?	—	—
I. Pick up a pea-sized crumb (Cheerio) easily with the *tips* of her thumb and a single finger		
(40w) (usually the 1st)?	—	—
J. Put a small toy down and take his hand off it, not just drop it?	—	—
(44w)		
K. Pick up a pea-sized crumb (Cheerio) easily with the tip of her thumb and a single finger		
(48w) (usually the 1st), without resting her arm or hand on the table while she is doing it? ...	—	—
L. Help you turn the pages of a book or magazine?	—	—
(52w) Throw a small ball with good casting motion?	—	—
M. Succeed in stacking 1 small toy such as a small block (1-inch) on top of a second one? ...	—	—
(56w)		
N. Succeed in stacking 3 small (1-inch) blocks?	—	—
(15m)		
O. Succeed in stacking 4 small (1-inch) blocks?	—	—
(18m) Turn pages of a book or magazine 2–3 at a time?	—	—

P. Succeed in stacking 6 small (1-inch) blocks? ....
(21m)

Q. Succeed in stacking 7 small (1-inch) blocks? ....
(24m) Thread the end of a shoelace through the hole at the end of a 1-inch safety pin? ....

R. Succeed in stacking 9 small (1-inch) blocks? ....
(30m) Turn pages in child's book 1 at a time? ....

S. Succeed in stacking 10 small (1-inch) blocks? ....
Hold a pencil or crayon with her fingers the way an adult does? ....
(36m) Try to cut with scissors, making the blades go up and down? ....

Group 4—(LANGUAGE BEHAVIOR)

DOES YOUR CHILD .... YES NO

A. Look vaguely at his surroundings, without definite focus? ....
(4w)

B. Make cooing sounds, "ooooo, aaaaaaah, oooooooooh?" ....
(8w)

C. Have the beginning of a laugh that does not quite come out? ....
(12w)

Group 4—(LANGUAGE BEHAVIOR, *continued*)

	YES	NO
DOES YOUR CHILD		
D. Laugh out loud?	—	—
(16w) Squeal by making her voice go up high?	—	—
E. Grunt, growl or make other deep-toned sounds, when he is not having a bowel movement? . . .		
(20w)	—	—
F. Turn to look at you if she doesn't see you, and you talk in a normal voice?		
(24w)	—	—
G. Make such sounds as da, ba, ka, or ga?	—	—
Imitate sounds you make by repeating them after you? (For example: a cough, tongue-click,		
(28w) razz)	—	—
H. Definitely combine 2 similar sounds, such as ba-ba, ga-ga, da-da, even though she doesn't		
mean anything by them?	—	
Respond to the tone of voice when you say "no-no" to her, although she may go ahead with		
(32w) what she was doing after pausing?	—	

A "WORD" IS A SOUND USED CONSISTENTLY TO MEAN A PERSON, OBJECT OR
GROUP OF OBJECTS

I. Say any 1 "word"?	—	—
(36w) Make noises in response to singing or music? (For example: la-la-la)	—	—

234

J. Say any 2 "words?" . . . . __ __

    Play any nursery games just if you ask her to, so you are sure she knows what the words mean?

(40w) Circle the ones she plays: bye-bye; pat-a-cake; peek-a-boo; so big . . . . __ __

K. Say any 3 "words?" . . . . __ __

    Follow any simple commands you give him, without your using gestures, such as "Come

(44w) here," "Sit down," "Put that down?" . . . . __ __

L. Say any 4 "words?" . . . . __ __

    Look at any of the *objects* around the house when you ask her to, without your pointing to

(48w) them or looking at them yourself, such as light, shoe, ball, TV? . . . . __ __

M. Say 6 "words?" . . . . __ __

(52w) Pat at, or try to pick up, large colored pictures in a book or magazine? . . . . __ __

N. Say 8 "words?" . . . . __ __

(56w) Go in to another room to get a familiar toy or object when you ask her to? . . . . __ __

How many words does he say? Please CIRCLE ONE: (9 or fewer), (10–19), (20–30), (30–50), (50 or more).

O. Point to 1 body part when you ask him to? . . . . __ __

(15m)

P. Combine 2–3 words which are different ideas, such as "Daddy bye," "Go car" (not "All right,"

    "What's this")? . . . . __ __

    Point to a picture just when you ask her to (for example: "Show me the dog"), without your

(18m) pointing or looking at it first? . . . . __ __

Group 4—(LANGUAGE BEHAVIOR, *continued*)

DOES YOUR CHILD .... YES   NO

Q. Name 1 picture in a book, just if you ask him? .... | | | |

Carry out the following directions, when you give them to him 1 at a time without pointing or
using gestures?

"Put the ball [or some other toy] on the table" .... | | | |

"Put the ball [or some other toy] on the chair" .... | | | |

"Give the ball [or some other toy] to mommy [or daddy]" .... | | | |

(21m) "Give the ball [or some other toy] to me" .... | | | |

R. Use pronouns such as "me, mine, I, you"? CIRCLE the ones used............................... | | | |

Make 3–4 word sentences? .... | | | |

Give example: _____

Name the following objects?   Point to the following objects if you name them?

	YES	NO			YES	NO
Ball				Ball		
Key				Key		
Pencil				Pencil		
Penny				Penny		

Point correctly in the attached pictures when you say, "Show me the baby sleeping; show me

(24m)   the baby eating?" .... | | | |

236

Carry out the following directions when you ask him to, without pointing or using gestures?
"Put the ball" (or other object you give him)

On the chair .... | | |
Under the chair .... | | |
In back of (behind) the chair .... | | |
(30m) In front of the chair .... | | |

T. Tell you what to do with the following objects? CIRCLE which ones: pencil, key, penny ... | |
Tell you her first and last name when you ask her? .... | |
Point to the correct colors when you ask her? CIRCLE which ones: red, yellow, blue,
(36m) green .... | |

Reference to the chart below will indicate the age-placement of the language patterns from 15–36 months. For ease of recording they have been grouped at a single age, but they are achieved over a spread of several adjacent ages.

Age in Months	15	18	21	24	30	36
# of Words	10–19	20–30	30–50	50+	++	++
# Directional commands	1	2	4	++	++	++
Pronouns	—	—	me, mine	I, you	++	++
Identifies # objects	—	2	4	++	++	++
Names # objects	—	1	3	4	++	++
Gives use # objects	—	—	—	—	1	2
# Prepositional commands	—	—	—	—	2	3
Identifies # colors	—	—	—	—	—	2

Group 5—(PERSONAL-SOCIAL BEHAVIOR)

DOES YOUR CHILD	YES	NO
A. Watch a person moving around the room?	—	—
(8w) Smile back at you if you just nod your head and talk to her?	—	—
B. Recognize his bottle when he sees it, before you put it in his mouth?	—	—
(12w) Hold his hand up and look at it?	—	—
C. Put both hands on her bottle when you are feeding her?	—	—
Smile and talk to herself when you put her *close* to a large mirror (dresser or bathroom cabinet	—	—
(16w) size)?	—	—
D. Lick at a toy he takes to his mouth?	—	—
(20w) Know the difference between strangers and people who belong in the house? . .	—	—
E. Get hold of her foot when she is lying on her back?	—	—
Reach out and pat her image when you put her *close* to a large mirror (dresser or bathroom	—	—
(24w) cabinet size)?	—	—
F. Put his foot in his mouth when he is lying on his back?	—	—
(28w) Bite and chew on his toys, not just lick at them?	—	—
G. Feed herself a cracker, taking definite bites until it is almost finished?	—	—
(32w) Take *milk*, not just water or juice, from a regular cup or glass if you hold it? . .	—	—
H. Hold his own bottle and pick it up again if it drops before he is finished?	—	—
Imitate nursery games if you do them first? CIRCLE which ones: bye-bye, pat-a-cake,	—	—
(36w) peek-a-boo, so big.	—	—

I. Hold a toy out to you but not let go of it in your hand unless you take it from her? . . . . —— ——
(40w) Help you when you dress her by pushing her arm through her sleeve once it is started in? . . . . —— ——

J. Release a toy into your hand if you hold out your hand and ask him for it? . . . . —— ——
(44w) Help you when you dress him by lifting his foot for his shoe or diaper? . . . . —— ——

K. Play ball *with* you, by rolling or throwing it to you? . . . . —— ——
(48w)

L. Indicate what he wants by pointing to it or looking at it, so you don't have to guess which one
of several things he wants? . . . . —— ——
(52w) Hug and kiss a doll or stuffed animal? . . . . —— ——

M. Feed himself part of his food *with a spoon*, although it may spill when he does it? . . . . —— ——
(15m) Pull you by the hand or clothes to show you some specific object or activity? . . . . —— ——

N. Handle a regular cup or glass well enough that she can drink from it and put it down without
tipping it over? . . . . —— ——
(18m) Imitate the things you do around the house, such as sweeping, dusting, hammering nails? . . . . —— ——

O. Use a fork to pick up his food and eat it? . . . . —— ——
(21m) Pretend to feed or dress a doll or stuffed animal? . . . . —— ——

P. Push a doll carriage or stroller with good steering and be able to back it out if she get stuck? . . . —— ——
(24m) Be allowed to carry breakables such as glasses or dishes? . . . . —— ——

Group 5—(PERSONAL-SOCIAL, *continued*)

DOES YOUR CHILD	YES	NO
Q. Pour well from 1 glass to another with very little spilling?	—	—
(30m) Put on a coat or jacket by himself, finding the armholes correctly?	—	—
R. Ask to go to the toilet during the day and stay dry most nights?	—	—
(36m) Get dressed by herself when you help with hard-to-reach fasteners?	—	—

Nursery Games are grouped at a single age for ease of recording, but are spread over several ages.

	Language*	Personal-Social†
32 w	—	Peek-a-boo
36 w	—	Any 2
40 w	Any 1	Any 3
44 w	Any 2	Any 3

*Language = performs on verbal request; knows meaning of words
† Personal-Social = imitates performance of someone else

240

APPENDICES

Appendix A
Procedures for the
Revision of the
Developmental
Schedules

THE SAMPLE

The sample used for revising the developmental schedules was drawn from the Albany area. It was a volunteer population solicited through local pediatricians, health clinics, and media publicity. Requests were made to all referral sources for "normal" infants who met the following criteria: delivery at term, within two weeks of the expected date of confinement; birth weight of 2500 grams or more; single birth; no developmental delays and no abnormalities.

All examinations occurred between January, 1975 and December, 1977. Children were examined at 4, 8, 12, 16, 20, 24, 28, 32, 36, 40, 44, 48, 52 and 56 weeks, and at 15, 18, 21, 24, 30 and 36 months. They were seen 3 days on either side of the "week" birthday. One week was allowed on either side of the "month" age. Because only major developmental abnormality could be observed at 4, 8, and 12 weeks, it was necessary to see an infant examined at one of these ages at a later age to insure that no minor developmental problems existed.

The total number of examinations completed was 1053, but only 927 were used in deriving the new schedules. A small percentage,

Table A–1. Mean Education for the Sample and for the Albany Area in 1975
Fathers and Mothers of Child-bearing Age

| | Sample | | | | | |
| | 4–56 weeks | | 15–36 months | | Albany Area | |
	No.*	Education	No.*	Education	No.	Education
Fathers	628	14.4	297	13.3	2803	12.7
Mothers	625	15.3	293	13.7	2596	13.5

*Number is number of examinations. There are no differences if number of children is used instead.

1.6%, could not be used because of behavior problems such as crying or acting up, and 3.7% were excluded because they had minor neuromotor abnormalities. 1.5% were our own errors in calculating the age of the child, 1.7% were infants seen at 4, 8, or 12 weeks who did not return for the required second examination, while 3.5% were children 15–36 months of age whose mothers had 14 or more years of education. They were discarded on a random basis to make the sample more representative of the Albany population and constituted 11% of the children in that age group.

This process of elimination was carried out because it became clear after the first 18 months of the study that the mean educational level of the mothers who volunteered was about 1.75 years higher than that of the mothers of child-bearing age in the Albany area population. Previous studies have shown that in the first year of life there are no significant differences in development based on sociocultural status.[7,10] In the sample examined up to that point there also were no significant differences in any area of behavior by maternal education at the infant ages. Consequently, no attempt was made to secure a more representative sample in the 4–56-week age range. Mothers with less education were secured for the 15–36-month age range, since it was not absolutely certain at what age prior to 3 years the sociocultural differences emerge.

Table A-1 shows the mean education for the sample and for the mothers of child-bearing age and the respective fathers for the 1975 births in the Albany area. The mean education for the fathers in the 15–36-month sample remains slightly higher than those of the Albany area. Table A-2 shows the distribution of the mothers' education for the sample by race. About 75% of the Black mothers have a high school education or less, while approximately 70% of the White mothers have at least some college. Of the total sample, 12% are

Table A–2. Distribution of Mother's Education by Race
Per Cent with Indicated Years Completed

Race	N	7–9	10–11	12	13–15	16	17+
White	781	1.2	5.8	25.0	27.9	20.6	19.5
Black	143	4.9	22.3	49.7	9.1	2.8	11.2

Black, the same as the percentage of Blacks in the Albany area and comparable to the national average. However, at ages 15–36 months, 20% of the sample are Black. The mean education of White mothers of child-bearing age in the Albany area is similar to that of the U.S. population; for the Blacks it is a little higher.

Table A-3 compares the 4–56-week and 15–36-month age groups on several demographic variables. As would be expected, the younger children are more often only children. The mean Hollingshead Index of Social Status for both ages is in the upper third. By design it is lower for the older children, as is the lower percentage of White children.

Table A–3. Selected Demographic Variables for Sample
by Age at Examination

	Age	
	4–56 weeks	15–36 months
Number of Examinations	630	297
Father's Age	29.4	29.9
Mother's Age	27.3	27.2
% Only Children	48	37
% Male	52.5	52.2
% White	87	79
Mean Birth Weight	3466	3404
Mean Gestation	281.4	281.5
Father's Hollingshead	33.1	41.9

EXAMINATION PROCEDURES

Approximately 1250 items were selected for evaluation, almost all of them from the original Gesell material. Where applicable, each behavior was evaluated with each of the test objects; for example, "transfers adeptly" could have occurred with any of the cubes, the bell, the ring-string or the cup. Some new items we devised and a few were adapted from other tests, although not necessarily evaluated in the same fashion. For example, uncovering and unwrapping a cube appear in the Bayley[1], inserting a string of beads into a tube in the Uzgiris and Hunt scales,[11] and several language items are in the REEL.[2]

Each examination was videotaped and the behavior recorded by an observer on the one of the seven recording sets which was appropriate for the age of the child. The examiner then recorded the observations on the original Gesell Developmental Schedules and assigned age levels in each area of behavior. All examinations were done by one of the three authors. When disagreements occurred about whether or not a particular behavior occurred, the videotape was reviewed to determine what actually happened and concordance was reached. Interobserver reliabilities for 48 independently recorded examinations are presented later.

Mean DQs by age at examination as well as a sample of individual item successes were examined for each of the 3 study years to see if there were any systematic changes of either acceleration or deceleration between the years. Fluctuations due to small sample sizes at individual ages did occur, but the direction of such fluctuations varied. The DQs in each area for each year for the total 4–56-week age group was virtually identical. For the 15–36-month age group, years 1 and 2 were the same, but year 3 was lower in adaptive and language behavior because of the deliberate attempt to include children whose mothers had less than a high school education.

AGE PLACEMENT OF BEHAVIOR PATTERNS

Of the total number of behaviors examined, 489 were selected for inclusion on the revised schedules: Adaptive behavior, 145; Gross Motor behavior, 98; Fine Motor behavior, 56; Language behavior, 109; Personal-Social behavior, 81. The criteria for placement of an item at a particular age were as follows: It must be achieved by 50% of the children at that age; it must be a behavior which either increases or decreases with age, or is a focal pattern which appears at a particular age and then disappears from the behavior repertoire; and it must distinguish between ages. Increasing patterns generally are those which become a permanent part of the child's behavior repertoire, even though they may undergo development and elaboration with increasing maturity. Decreasing or focal patterns generally are those which are temporary in nature because they are replaced by more mature patterns at later ages.

Some examples of patterns in different areas are tabulated as illustrations of the method used. The behavior patterns and the percentages of children demonstrating the behavior at the indicated ages are shown. The age placement of the behavior is boxed.

Increasing patterns

Takes a large fraction of weight supported around chest:

Age	8w	12w	16w	20w	24w	28w	32w	36w
%	4	11	36	54	74	91	96	98

Plays pat-a-cake:

Age	28w	32w	36w	40w	44w	48w
%	6	34	36	69	86	82

Spontaneous scribble:

Age	52w	56w	15m	18m	21m
%	10	14	52	82	96

Dumps pellet spontaneously:

Age	52w	56w	15m	18m	21m
%	2	6	22	62	80

Follows 2 directional commands:

Age	56w	15m	18m	21m
%	2	20	64	88

Throws ball overhand:

Age	24m	30m	36m
%	12	44	62

Gives full name:

Age	24m	30m	36m
%	6	40	59

Decreasing and Focal Patterns

Decreasing and focal patterns usually are interrelated and show the shifts as the more mature permanent pattern replaces the immature one. Examples of three related patterns:

	Age	4w	8w	12w	16w
TONIC-NECK-REFLEX PREDOMINATES	%	92	46	4	—
SYMMETRIC POSTURES SEEN	%	37	79	96	—
SYMMETRIC POSTURES PREDOMINATE	%	4	14	82	94

	Age	20w	24w	28w	32w	36w	40w	44w	48w
PALMAR GRASP	%	26	86	60	36	10	—	—	—
RADIAL PALMAR GRASP	%	4	32	81	96	78	47	31	18
RADIAL DIGITAL GRASP	%	—	—	6	28	50	78	91	90

An example of one decreasing pattern and its related increasing pattern:

	Age	4w	8w	12w	16w	20w	24w
COMPLETE HEAD LAG	%	92	64	11	—	—	—
NO HEAD LAG	%	—	—	4	42	76	84

An example of a focal pattern which is replaced by a more mature pattern:

	Age	16w	20w	24w	28w	32w	36w	40w	44w	48w
BANGS BELL	%	—	26	38	56	76	48	49	30	14
WAVES BELL	%	—	—	—	17	34	44	73	80	76

Several patterns which were on the original schedules did not meet the criteria, either because they did not distinguish between adjacent ages or were not exhibited by 50% at any age. They and the remaining patterns which did not meet the criteria were discarded.

For example:

	Age	24w	28w	32w	36w	40w	44w	48w
HOLDS RING, MANIPULATES STRING	%	6	25	42	38	46	38	22
GRASPS 3RD CUBE	%	—	23	18	10	24	18	—

When a behavior could have occurred in more than one situation, without necessarily achieving 50% in any single situation, the individual patterns were summarized. For each age the percentage of children achieving in one, two or "n" situations was listed. In the case of "transfers adeptly," the data are shown by age for infants not achieving and the opposite, those achieving in one or more situations, such as with any of the cubes, the cup, the bell or the ring-string.

	Age	20w	24w	28w	32w	36w	40w
NOT ACHIEVING	%	92	68	15	4	8	4
ACHIEVING IN ONE OR MORE SITUATIONS	%	8	32	85	96	92	96

VALIDATING THE AGE PLACEMENTS

After all the age placements of the behaviors had been made, tentative new schedules were constructed for each of the 20 ages. The data for each of the 927 examinations were transferred to these tentative schedules and age levels assigned in each area for each child. The purpose was to determine if the new schedules assigned maturity ages appropriate for the chronologic age of the child. If any mean age was statistically outside the 95% confidence limits, the behavior patterns for each case were reviewed to determine if any errors had been made and adjustments were undertaken. Some reassignments of age placements were done after this review. Interscorer reliabilities derived from independent assignments of these age levels are presented later.

Table A-4 lists the mean DQs and SDs for each age in each area of behavior. All the quotients at 4, 8 and 12 weeks are too high; modification could not be accomplished. For example, "symmetric postures predominate" was placed at 12 weeks where 82% accomplished the behavior, not at 8 weeks where 14% accomplished it.

Table A–4. Revised Developmental Quotients
Means and Standard Deviations by Age at Examination

Age of Behavior	Age	4w	8w	12w	16w	20w	24w	28w	32w	36w	40w	44w	48w	52w	56w	15m	18m	21m	24m	30m	36m†
	No.	24	28	28	50	50	50	52	50	50	50	50	50	50	50	50	50	50	50	50	47
ADAPTIVE	Mean	128	102	109	103	104	103	98	101	98	100	101	100	99	98	100	102	100	101	99	103
	S.D.	41	19	13	11	13	9	9	10	9	6	7	8	16	6	10	9	8	12	11	16
GROSS MOTOR	Mean	163	120	108	106*	100	99	101	99	103	104	101	100	102	104	104	100	100	103	100	97
	S.D.	55	17	17	14	12	10	13	12	13	11	9	8	18	10	10	11	9	12	13	10
FINE MOTOR	Mean	159	112	107	98	99	99	99	100	98	101	102	99	100	99	102	101	100	106*	101	92*
	S.D.	53	21	19	13	13	10	10	9	9	8	7	7	17	12	11	11	13	14	12	10
LANGUAGE	Mean	128	118	105	105*	105	101	103	97	98	101	101	96	101	101	97	99	98	98	98	97
	S.D.	40	30	11	15	16	8	8	7	11	9	10	11	17	9	10	13	12	16	14	14
PERSONAL-SOCIAL	Mean	137	112	104	107*	104	101	103*	102	97	100	98	96*	101	98	101	104	101	102	100	103
	S.D.	46	18	16	15	14	10	6	9	8	6	7	5	16	8	11	7	7	11	11	9

*Outside the 95% Confidence Limits, above ages 4, 8 and 12 weeks
†Asymptotic quotients obtained; no children over 36 months were examined

Table A–5. Revised Developmental Quotients by Mother's Education
Means and Standard Deviations, Ages 15–36 Months

Age	Mother's Educ.	No.	Adaptive Mean	S.D.	Gross Motor Mean	S.D.	Fine Motor Mean	S.D.	Language Mean	S.D.	Personal-Social Mean	S.D.
15m	12–	22	102	11	105	8	103	14	99	12	101	10
	13+	28	98	10	102	10	102	9	97	9	101	10
18m	12–	23	100	9	101	9	102	10	94	12	100	6
	13+	27	102	10	101	12	101	13	103	12	108	6
									p<.02		p<.001	
21m	12–	31	99	9	100	10	99	14	97	12	101	7
	13+	19	102	8	99	9	101	12	100	13	101	8
24m	12–	26	98	13	104	13	104	14	94	15	103	13
	13+	24	104	10	103	10	108	15	103	16	102	10
									p<.05			
30m	12–	32	97	11	102	14	99	12	96	13	100	12
	13+	18	101	11	104	11	102	12	104	14	99	10
									p<.05			
36m	12–	25	97	16	99	11	92	11	90	12	103	9
	13+	22	109	14	95	8	91	8	104	12	102	8
			p<.001						p<.001			

In addition, 1 or 2 weeks at these ages represent a significantly greater proportion of the infant's life span than they do at later ages. Assigning a maturity level of 5 weeks to a 4-week old already gives a DQ of 125. Behavior at these ages we find to be very amorphous, dependent on physiologic state, and evaluated quite subjectively. Maturity levels must be taken with several grains of salt. These ages are included primarily for rough evaluation of an older infant with developmental delay. The behavior is not predictive of later development in normal infants. Of the remaining 85 means, 7, or 8%, are outside the confidence limits, 3 of them at 16 weeks of age.

The mean DQs were calculated separately by maternal education: high school or less and at least some college. Among the 60 mean DQs from 16 weeks to 15 months, 2 are statistically significantly different, in favor of those with less maternal education. Overall, the direction of the differences varies.

Table A-5 presents the mean DQs and SDs for 15–36 months for each of the maternal education groups. Significantly greater language DQs for the higher maternal education group start at 18 months. The adaptive DQs are not significantly higher until 36 months. Golden, *et al*,[5] in 1971 also reported no significant differences in measures of intellectual development by maternal education or by other indices of social status, in a group of Black children, until 3 years of age.

Since the sample was an all-volunteer one, accusations could be made that mothers would enroll their children in the study only if they thought they were "very bright." To obviate this possibility infants were enrolled before 6 weeks of age, from the start of the investigation. There were 233 such infants, almost all enrolled right after delivery. The mean adaptive DQ was 103 for this group, compared to 100 for the remainder of the children.

RELIABILITIES

Interobserver reliability was evaluated in two different areas. The percentage of agreement between observers for individual items was determined on a sample of 48 cases, covering the age range from 16 weeks to 21 months. The overall percentage of agreement for 305 individual behavior patterns and 2302 comparisons was 93.7%, as shown in Table A-6. It varied from 88% in Fine Motor behavior to 97% in Language.

Table A–6. Interobserver Reliability for Behavior Patterns
Ages 16 weeks to 21 months

Area of Behavior	No. of Items	No. of Comparisons	Per Cent Agreement
ADAPTIVE	92	826	92
GROSS MOTOR	66	450	96
FINE MOTOR	30	263	88
LANGUAGE	48	354	97
PERSONAL-SOCIAL	69	409	95
TOTAL	305	2302	93.7

Table A-7. Interrater Reliability for Assigning Maturity Age Levels

Age	No. of Cases	Adaptive	Gross Motor	Fine Motor	Language	Personal-Social
4w	24	.93	.93	.84	.98	.96
16w	20	.97	.96	.96	.98	.97
24w	20	.93	.96	.97	.95	.97
40w	20	.88	.99	.87	.98	.94
48w	20	.96	.98	.93	.99	.93
52w	20	.92	.99	.99	.98	*—
18m	20	.93	.94	*—	.99	.95
24m	20	.99	.97	*—	.99	.95
36m	20	.98	.98	.98	.98	.96

*Levels not assigned independently

In a second procedure, one of the authors assigned age levels on the new schedules for all children at each age; a second author selected a sample of 20 from the beginning, middle, and end of each age group. Pearson r values were calculated for 184 of the cases at 4, 16, 24, 40, 48 and 52 weeks and 18, 24 and 36 months. Disagreement between the two evaluators was discussed and adjusted *after* the calculations were completed. Table A-7 shows that the r values ranged from .84 to .99. There were 73% between .95 and .99, 20% between .90 and .94, and 6.6% between .84 and .89.

Previous studies have shown that pediatric residents with little training can do an evaluation and assign DQs with similar high rates of reliability.[6]

Table A–8. Comparison of the Original Age-Placement of Behavior Patterns with the Revised Age-Placement

Adaptive Behavior

Cube, Cup and Cubes Behavior

Age in Weeks	Original Placement	Revised Placement
32		Hits, pushes cube with cube
		Removes cube from cup
36	Hits, pushes cube with cube	
	Hits cube against cup	Hits cube against cup
40	Fingers cube in cup	
	Matches 2 cubes	Matches 2 cubes
44	Removes cube from cup	
	Cube into cup, no release	Cube into cup, no release
		Uncovers cube
48	Sequential play	Releases 2 cubes into cup
52	Releases cube into cup	

THE CHANGES

Differences between the original and the revised developmental schedules are compared by noting both the average change in DQs and the difference in the age placement of individual behavior patterns, as well as any change in the developmental sequences.

In *adaptive behavior* the DQs assigned on the original schedules average 110; behavior is achieved about 10% earlier by today's infants and children. The sequences of behavioral acquisition in this area have remained almost entirely unaltered. For example, in the 24–48-week age range, most of the sequences are the same. Some of them have changed; two are listed at top of next page.

Sequences the same:

APPROACH: 2-hand approach (24 w) — — — — →1-hand approach (28w)

MASSED CUBES: Grasps 2 (24 w) — — — — →grasps 2 more than momentarily (28w) — — — — →grasps 2 prolongedly (32w)

CUP AND CUBES: Retains cube, regards cup (24w) — — — — →retains cube, grasps cup (28w) — — — — →hits cube against cup (36w) — — — — →cube into cup without release (44w) — — — — →releases 2 cubes into cup (48w)

PELLET AND BOTTLE: Holds bottle, grasps pellet (36w) — — — — →points at pellet through glass (40w) — — — — →tries to insert pellet (48w) — — — — →inserts pellet (52w)

Sequences different:

PELLET AND BOTTLE: Regards pellet if it drops out (32w) before holds bottle and grasps pellet (36w)

Approaches and grasps pellet first (44w and 48w) after holds bottle and grasps pellet (36w)

Tables A-8, A-9, and A-10 demonstrate the alteration in the age of acquisition of skills.

Table A–9. Comparison of the Original Age-Placement of Behavior Patterns with the Revised Age-Placement

Adaptive Behavior

Pellet and Bottle Behavior

Age in weeks	Original Placement	Revised Placement
32		Regards pellet if drops out
36		Index finger approach
		Holds bottle, grasps pellet
40	Regards pellet if drops out	Points at pellet through glass
	Index finger approach	
	Holds bottle, grasps pellet	
	Approaches pellet first	
44	Points at pellet through glass	Approaches pellet first

Table A–10. Comparison of the Original Age-Placement of Behavior Patterns with the Revised Age-Placement

Adaptive Behavior

Bell, Ring-String Behavior

Age in weeks	Original Placement	Revised Placement
40	Grasps by handle ⟶	Grasps by handle
	Waves ⟶	Waves
		Regards, pokes clapper
		Sees connection between ring and string
44	Regards, pokes clapper	
	Sees connection between ring and string	

In *gross motor behavior* there has been an acceleration of approximately 17% and somewhat greater alteration in sequencing, as illustrated by the following sequences.

Sequences the same:

Stands hands held (28w) – – – –→stands holding rail (32w) – – – –→pulls to feet at rail (36w) – – – –→walks 2 hands held (44w) – – – –→walks 1 hand held (48w) – – – –→rises independently (52w).

Sits well, leaning on hands (24w) – – – –→sits erect about 1 minute (28w) – – – –→sits steady 10+ minutes (32w) – – – –→sits indefinitely steady (36w)

Sequences different:

Cruises at the railing (40w) now earlier than walks both hands held (44w)

Stands alone (48w) now the same as walks 1 hand held (48w)

Squats in play (56w) now before walks alone, runs, climbs stairs

Climbs into adult chair (56w) now before walks alone, seldom falls, runs, climbs stairs

Climbs into small chair (52w) is defined differently from seats self in small chair (previously 18 months)

Tables A-11 and A-12 indicate that all of the behavior patterns at 36–56 weeks in gross motor behavior have shifted to lower ages, in contrast to adaptive behavior where some of the items have retained their original age placement.

Table A–11. Comparison of the Original Age-Placement of Behavior Patterns with the Revised Age-Placement

Gross Motor Behavior

Standing Behavior

Age in weeks	Original Placement	Revised Placement
36		Pulls to feet
		Lifts, replaces foot at rail
40	Pulls to feet	Cruises using 2 hands
		Retrieves toy from floor
		Lets self down with control
44	Lifts, replaces foot at rail	Walks, both hands held
		Cruises using 1 hand
48	Cruises	Walks, 1 hand held
	Walks, both hands held	Stands momentarily alone
		Few steps from object to object
52	Walks, 1 hand held	Picks up object from floor
56	Stands momentarily alone	

Table A–12. Comparison of the Original Age-Placement of Behavior Patterns with the Revised Age-Placement

Gross Motor Behavior

Sitting, Prone Behavior

Age in weeks	Original Placement	Revised Placement
36		Sits indefinitely steady
		Goes to prone
		Creeps
		Prone to sitting
40	Sits indefinitely steady	
	Goes to prone	
	Creeps	
44		Pivots in sitting
48	Pivots in sitting	

There has been no change in the sequencing in *fine motor be-havior*. The developmental rate has remained essentially unchanged at the younger ages, but there has been a slight acceleration of 5% at 56 weeks to 36 months because tower building has been accomplished earlier. However, there are quite a few new items in the second and third years of life, providing a broader base for evaluating fine motor behavior at these ages. At the younger ages, grasps of pellet and string have been separated, and crude release has moved from 40 to 44 weeks.

In *language behavior* the acceleration has averaged about 12%. There has been the addition of several new items, but the chief changes have been in separating behaviors which previously were combined, and making a greater differentiation between expressive and receptive language. There are now language items at 44 and 48 weeks as a result of the separation and a more precise counting of words used. Tables A-13 and A-14 show the 32–48-week age range.

Table A–13. Comparison of the Original Age-Placement of Behavior Patterns with the Revised Age-Placement

Expressive Language

Age in weeks	Original Placement	Revised Placement
36	Da-da or equivalent (*e.g.*, ma-ma) ——→	Ma-ma as sound
		— — — — — — — — —
		1 "word"
		— — — — — — — — —
		Sings along with music
40	1 "word"	
	— — — — — — — — —	
	"Dada" with meaning ——→	"Dada" with meaning
	— — — — — — — — —	
	"Mama" with meaning	
44		"Mama" with meaning
		— — — — — — — — —
		Any 3 "words"
48		Any 4 "words"
52	2 "words" besides "mama" and "dada"	

Table A–14. Comparison of the Original Age-Placement of Behavior Patterns with the Revised Age-Placement

Receptive Language

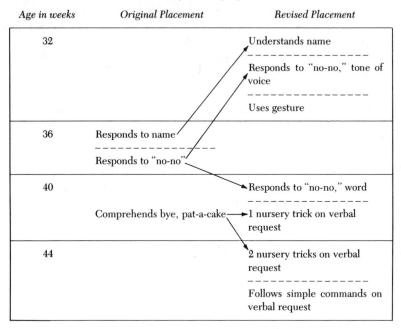

Age in weeks	Original Placement	Revised Placement
32		Understands name
		Responds to "no-no," tone of voice
		Uses gesture
36	Responds to name	
	Responds to "no-no"	
40		Responds to "no-no," word
	Comprehends bye, pat-a-cake	1 nursery trick on verbal request
44		2 nursery tricks on verbal request
		Follows simple commands on verbal request

In *personal-social behavior* there has been an acceleration of approximately 16%. A few scattered items retain their original placement, but most of the behavior has shifted to lower age levels. Personal-social behavior is almost all based on historical information. However, in the other areas history and observations have agreed. There is little reason to assume that the mothers are overreporting only in the personal-social area.

Appendix B
Materials

EXAMINATION MATERIALS

The materials for the developmental examination are simple, and are pictured in Figures B-1 and B-2. Some can be secured or improvised readily. However, care should be taken not to use objects which are markedly different from those prescribed in dimensions, texture and appearance, since weight and size do influence an infant's ability to handle them. The materials are being distributed by Nigel Cox, 69 Fawn Drive, Cheshire, CT 06410.

The following materials are needed for carrying out the examination:

- Audubon Bird Call (available from bird supply stores or catalogs)
- Ball, large: 4–6 inches in diameter
- Ball, small: 2½-inch diameter
- Beads and Tube: 18-inch-long string of beads which cannot be compacted sufficiently to fit into the tube in a handful; tube which cannot stand on its own and holds the length of beads if they are dropped in lengthwise.
- Bell: 3 inches high with wooden handle, and metal bowl 1½ inches in diameter
- Big and Little Block: 1-inch block and 1½-inch block of the same color.
- Bottle, clear glass: 2½ inches high, mouth 1-inch diameter
- Catbells: 3 metal bells on shower-curtain ring

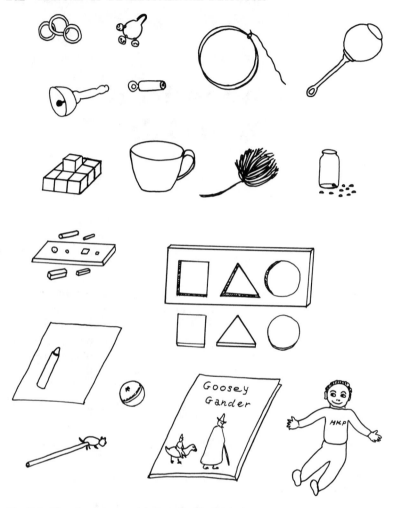

Fig. B-1. Examination materials described in the text.

- Color Forms and Card: 8½ by 11 inches with 5 forms and matching cutouts, red. Circle, 2-inch diameter; square, 2-inch sides; triangle, 2⅝-inch sides; semicircle, 3¼-inch diameter; cross, 2⅞ inches long, ¹⁵⁄₁₆-inch-wide arms
- Colors: small red, yellow, blue, and green blocks or other items

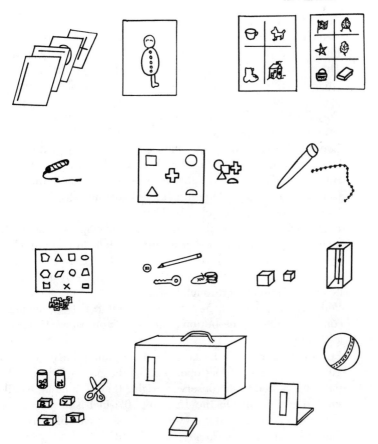

Fig. B-2. Examination materials described in the text.

- Crayons: Staonal #2 marking crayon, 5 inches long, ½-inch diameter
- Cubes: 10 red, 1-inch edges, squared corners, made of hard wood
- Cup: aluminum, 12-ounce capacity, 3¾-inch top diameter, 2¼ inches high
- Doll: small, unbreakable, clear features
- Forms for Drawing: set of 5-inch by 8-inch cards with form in heavy black outline ¹⁄₁₆-inch wide. Circle, cross, square and triangle: 3 inches for diameter, length, or sides; horizontal

line, 4 inches; vertical line, 7 inches; rectangle with diagonals, 4 inches by 2¾ inches; diamond, 2¼ inches each side

- Formboard, Three-hole: ½-inch board, 6 inches by 14 inches. Three holes equidistant from each other and from edges; circle, 3½-inch diameter; triangle, 3¾-inch sides; square, 3¹/₁₆-inch sides
- Formboard Blocks: contrasting color ⅞ inches thick. Circle, 3⅜ inches; triangle, 3⅝ inches; square, 2¹⁵/₁₆ inches
- Loud and Soft: two opaque plastic pill containers with tight-fitting lids, one containing thumb tacks, the other containing cut scraps of film (or any substances of approximately the same weight which can be differentiated as loud and soft)
- Paper: onionskin, 8½ inches by 11 inches
- Pegboard: ¾-inch board 3 inches wide and approximately 12 inches long with holes cut just large enough to accommodate two pairs of pegs: large round ⅜-inch and small round ¼-inch diameter; large square ⅜-inch and small square ¼-inch sides; holes cut completely through board
- Pellets: edible (sugar), 5–8 mm in diameter; flat on one side, convex on other (shoe-button penny candy on paper strips now available)
- Performance Box (or Basket of similar dimensions): 15¾ by 10¼ by 7½ inches. The open end of the box is 10¼ by 7½; with this placed to the observer's right, there is a metal handle for lifting on top. On the 15¾- by 10¼-inch side facing the observer is a vertical slot 3 by 1⅛ inches which will accommodate the square block from the formboard.
- Picture Book: Goosey Gander, a variety of nursery rhymes, or any child's book which has common objects such as hat, shoe, dog, baby, and common situations, such as eating, sleeping, and playing ball.
- Picture Card (a): dog, shoe, cup, house
- Picture Card (b): clock, basket, book, flag, leaf, star
- Rattle: 6 inches long; bowl, 2¼-inch diameter with slender handle, ⅜-inch diameter
- Ring-string: wooden, red, 4-inch diameter; 10-inch string, 2-mm diameter
- Safety Pin and Shoelace: 1-inch safety pin, stiff shoelace with round tip that just fits eye of safety pin
- Scissors: child's blunt end

- Test Objects: ball, examiner's shoe, key, pencil, penny
- Toy and Stick: toy, pipe cleaner fashioned to look like a dog approximately 1 inch by 2 inches; stick, 8-inch dowel, ¼-inch diameter
- Tricolored Rings: plaques on chain, interlocking rings, etc
- Up and Down Box: open-faced rectangular box, approximately 7 by 3 inches, with a bead on a string which is stretched vertically between the ends. Bead must move easily on string but be tight enough to stay in a placed position. Alternatively, any method of stretching a string to 7 inches
- Vertical Slot: plastic, 8 inches high by 4 inches wide, mounted on contrasting color 4- by 3½-inch base with vertical rectangular slot 3 by 1⅛ inches for insertion of square block from the formboard
- Yarn: pom-pom, 3-inch diameter on a 12-inch string

Additional items which are part of the Stanford-Binet test or the Merrill-Palmer test include:
Action Agents
Geometric Forms: card and matching forms
Incomplete man drawing

Special clinical equipment is described in Appendix B.

Picture books, cups, rattles, crayons and small plastic bottles can be purchased in local stores. Pellet substitutes must be firm as well as edible; cinnamon red-hots are satisfactory, but raisins and baby aspirin are contra-indicated. Multicolored cubes and natural wood rings are available in quantity from the following sources (1979 prices):

1-inch colored cubical blocks—$10.96/100
Ideal School Supply Company
11000 Lavergne Avenue
Oaklawn, Illinois 60453
Hold-Tite 4-inch wooden embroidery hoops—$4.60/dozen
Gibbs Manufacturing Company
606 Sixth Street, N.E.
Canton, Ohio 44702
The following items are obtainable on the open market:
Child's kindergarten table
Child's kindergarten chairs
Mirror (attach roller shade)

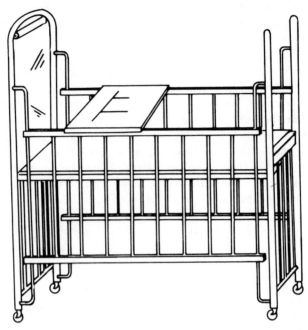

Fig. B-3. Clinical crib showing platform, tabletop 18 inches deep on adjustable side panels, roller shade covering mirror and end panel removed, with wooden box made to measure covering residual spikes.

SPECIAL CLINICAL EQUIPMENT

Clinical Crib. A hospital crib (30″ × 54″) with side panels adjustable by means of a hand-operated catch at the base of the panel is modified slightly, as shown in Figure B-3. Additional panel heights are provided by drilling extra holes in the upright rods on which the side panels ride. A sturdy wooden platform is used instead of a mattress; it may replace the springs entirely if desired. The foot-end panel is sawed off to provide a clearer view of the infant in the crib. The short spikes which are the remnants of the foot railings are capped with a wooden cover made to measure. An ingenious machine shop can remove the foot corner uprights while still permitting the side panels to be raised and lowered. If this is done, the view of the infant is entirely unobstructed.

Side view

3 screws ½"
apart; lowest
2½" above
side piece

8¼"

2 screws each side,
¾" from front edge,
½" down & apart

4½" |← 5¾" →|← 7¼" →|

|← 13" →|

Front View

2"

8¼"   6"

4½"

|← 7¾" →|

About ⁵⁄₈" by ⁵⁄₈"

Back view of
chair cover.
Top slips over
upright;
button holes
hook over
screws at front

Oblique View

2 bars in
back

Bars curved to allow
for back; center of
curve about $1^1/_8$" back from
front plane of upright

¾" wood

1 bar in front, at
bottom

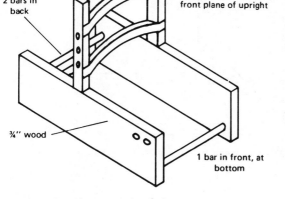

Fig. B-4. Plans for infant examining chair.

267

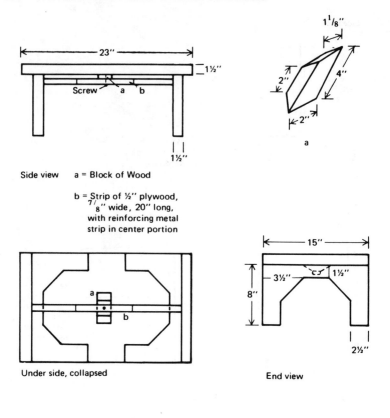

Side view   a = Block of Wood

b = Strip of ½" plywood,
⅞" wide, 20" long,
with reinforcing metal
strip in center portion

Under side, collapsed

End view

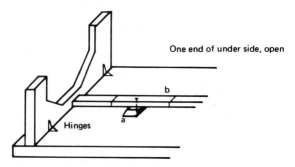

One end of under side, open

Fig. B-5. Plans for portable examining table, made of ¾-inch plywood.

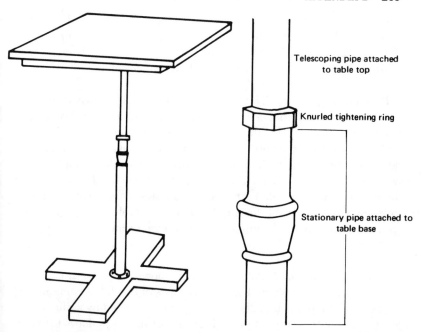

Telescoping pipe attached to table top

Knurled tightening ring

Stationary pipe attached to table base

Fig. B-6. Adjustable clinical examining table, showing details of plumber's pipe joint used to regulate height.

A mirror, large enough to cover completely the head-end panel of the crib, is fastened securely in place and a roller shade attached. The test objects are kept most conveniently in a shoe bag hung on the back of the crib head. A four-tier bag may be purchased and one row of pockets modified to hold the formboard and picture book.

The tabletop is sturdy plywood 18 inches deep, the width fitted to the crib size. Strips of quarter-round on the short edges hold it in place on top of the crib side rails while permitting it to slide back and forth freely.

Infant Examining Chair. The construction of the chair is indicated in Figure B-4. The chair is provided with a removable washable cover of canvas weight; it slips over the top of the chair back, slings forward loosely and hooks over the pairs of screws at the front of the side panels. The infant is secured in place with a broad canvas band around his chest. Several buttonholes are made in each side of the band to fit over one of the screws on the side uprights and allow adjustment. For the infant unable to sit alone, the chest band must be tight enough to provide firm support and prevent any slumping, so that the arms can be used freely. Usually this is at least one buttonhole tighter than you think would be comfortable.

Portable Test Table. This table's construction is shown in Figure B-5. In the event that a hospital crib with more than two panel heights is not available, the portable test table replaces the sliding tabletop, and the other procedures remain unchanged. The indicated height has been found adaptable for children of all sizes on a hospital ward. For very small infants, the entire chair is elevated on a suitable number of folded sheets or blankets. For the older infant who sits independently but is still too short to reach the tabletop properly, the chest band is fastened loosely merely to prevent him from getting out of the chair accidentally.

Adjustable Clinical Table. This table is shown in Figure B-6. It has a plywood top 2 by 3 feet. The stem consists of two telescoping metal pipes attached to metal plates. The height is regulated by a plumber's joint on the outer pipe. The base is cross bars of two-by-fours to allow room for comfortable foot placement. This table is used (1) for conducting the interview with the parents; (2) for the situations when the mother must hold the child, *e.g.*, the infant who will not leave her, the toddler too old for the crib but too small for the kindergarten chair, the handicapped child too big or too impaired for the infant examining chair; and (3) in conjunction with an adult chair, as a substitute for kindergarten furniture for the older child.

Appendix C
Audiovisual Aids

While audiovisual aids are not essential, an audiovisual record of infants and children in action provides something for which no number of words can substitute. We have not yet been able to revise the films which were prepared in the past and which supplemented the Third Edition of Developmental Diagnosis. *For those who would like to use it, however, one of these films illustrates all the adaptive, fine motor and gross motor patterns from 4 weeks to 15 months, and some up to 36 months, which appeared on the original Gesell Developmental Schedules. It must be viewed with caution, since confusion could be caused by the differing age-placements of the behavior patterns which reflect current behavior. Nevertheless, it could be a useful adjunct. A description of this film and the source for obtaining it follows.*

DEVELOPMENTAL EVALUATION IN INFANCY

Part I. Normal Adaptive and Fine Motor Behavior

A single pattern on the 15-month developmental schedule, inserting the pellet into the bottle, is selected as a culminating pattern, and the evolution of each of 7 patterns which must be integrated for its accomplishment is traced from age 4 weeks. The 7 patterns are ocular regard, active grasp, the development of approach, manipulation of the small object, interest in multiple objects, the concept of container and contained, and the development of voluntary release. In the course of demonstrating their synthesis, essentially all the adaptive and fine motor patterns on the developmental schedules between 4 weeks and 15 months are illustrated. The film then indicates how principles involved in the evolution of this culminating pattern can be applied to the evolution of more advanced patterns, by tracing tower building from 52 weeks to 3 years of age.

Part II. Normal Gross Motor Behavior

A similar 15-month culminating pattern, assuming the erect posture unassisted and walking independently, is traced in the same fashion. The integration of 6 patterns is followed from age 4 weeks to 15 months: head control, static; head control, dynamic; sitting, static; early locomotion, dynamic; standing, static; and standing, dynamic. The further evolution of the bipedal pattern is shown, and its relationship to cognitive behavior and the significance of a developmental approach are summarized briefly.

The film is 16-mm black-and-white optical sound, and is accompanied by a copy of the complete sound track. It may be purchased or rented by addressing inquiries to The Department of Photography and Cinema, The Ohio State University, 156 West 19th Avenue, Columbus, Ohio 43210.

The rental fee is $12.50. The purchase price for Part I, 1500 feet (42 minutes), is $145; Part II, 650 feet (18 minutes), $85; both parts $220.

References

1. Bayley N: Manual for the Bayley Scales of Infant Development. New York, The Psychological Corporation, 1969
2. Bzoch KR, League R: Receptive-Expressive Emergent Language Scale. Gainesville, The Tree of Life Press, 1970
3. Frankenburg, WK, Goldstein A, Camp BW: The revised Denver Developmental Screening Test. Its accuracy as a screening instrument. J Pediatr, 79: 988, 1971
4. Frankenburg, WK, van Doornick WJ, Liddell TN, Dick NP: The Denver Pre-screening Developmental Questionnaire (PDQ). Pediatrics 57: 744, 1976
5. Golden M, Birns B, Bridger W, Moss A: Social class differentiation in cognitive development among Black preschool children. Child Devel 42: 37, 1971
6. Knobloch H, Pasamanick B (eds): Gesell and Amatruda's Developmental Diagnosis, 3rd ed. Hagerstown, Harper & Row, 1974
7. Knobloch H, Pasamanick B: An evaluation of the consistency and predictive value of the 40-week Gesell developmental schedule. In Shagass C, Pasamanick B, (eds): Child Development and Child Psychiatry. Psychiatric Research Reports 13. Washington, Am Psych Assn, 1960, pp 10–31
8. Knobloch H, Stevens F, Malone A, Ellison P, Risemberg H: The validity of parental reporting of infant development. Pediatrics 63: 872, 1979
9. Malone A, Knobloch H, Stevens F, Ellison P, Risemberg H: Problems assessing outcome of neonatal intensive care (Unpublished data) 1977
10. Pasamanick B: A comparative study of the behavioral development of Negro infants. J Genet Psychol 69: 3, 1946
11. Uzgiris IC, Hunt JM: Assessment in Infancy. Ordinal Scales of Psychological Development. Urbana, University of Illinois Press, 1975

Index

Page numbers followed by the letter "t" indicate tabular material; those followed by "f" indicate illustrations.

277